Heal Thyself

for Health and Longevity

Queen Afua

EWORLD INC.

Buffalo, New York
14209
eeworldinc@yahoo.com

NOTICE

This book is intended as a reference volume only, not as a medical text. The information provided herein is designed to help you make informed decisions about your health. It is not intended to be a substitute for any treatment that may have been prescribed by your doctor. It is sold with the understanding that the publisher is not engaged in rendering medical advice. If you have a medical problem, we urge you to seek competent medical help.

 EWorld Inc.
Buffalo, New York 14209
eeworldinc@yahoo.com

Cover Illustration: Mshindo I.

Principal Editor:
Rhea Mandulo
Contributing Editor:
Sababu N. Plata
Assistant Editors:
Carol Daugherty, Shirley McRae, Gerianne F. Scott, Naikyemi S. B. Odedefaa (Cheryl J. Sneed), Hru Ankh Ra Semajh Se Ptah and Princess.

Photographs: Anthony Mills unless otherwise indicated.

Library of Congress Cataloging-in-Publication Data

Afua, Queen
  Heal Thyself for health and longevity/ Queen Afua
        p.   cm.
  Includes index.

  ISBN 978-1-61759-039-9

  1. Naturopathy.   2. Spiritual healing   3. Longevity   4. Fasting-Health
  aspects.   5. Self-care Health.   I. Title.
  RZ440.A36   98-
  14248154.6' 3--dc21615.5—dc21   CIP

Formally published by
A&B Publishers Group
Brooklyn, New York
ISBN 978-1-886433-76-3

                21 22   9 8
    Printed and Bound in the United States of America

Heal Thyself

Heal Thyself Declaration of Independence

"...I have the power to create in my life what I want and need. Purification of mind, body, and spirit is the key. Within this natural way of living and being, I choose not to cut, nor radiate, or drug my dis-ease away. Instead, I wash, pray, fast, juice and bless my dis-ease away."

EWORLD INC.

Buffalo, New York
14209
eeworldinc@yahoo.com

Contents

Preface

THE HEALER DIFFERS from the medical doctor in that the medical doctor is a learned and trained technician in methods for alleviating symptoms of illness that may or may not be part of his/her personal experience. The healer is someone who has through his/her personal experience learned to utilize life's obstacles for growth and development. When, through understanding trial and error, an obstacle, problem or illness is overcome and a new experience of benefit is born—out of an old problem, true healing has taken place.

When such an individual extends his/her healing experience to others to help guide them through what has been experienced, a healer is created. The process is continual. As the healer helps to guide others, he/she, too, is guided from within on the path of evolution.

In 1979, I had the pleasure to meet such an individual in the person of Queen Afua. A year later, I was to witness the opening of the Heal Thyself Natural Living and Education Center.

Since that time, she has been my mentor and inspiration on the journey to health. Through the years, I have been irrigated, steamed, bathed, 'herbed,' fasted and clay-packed by Queen Afua.

Presently, I can testify that the most powerful healing agent of this 'extra' ordinary person is Queen Afua herself.

At the time of this writing, I have had the pleasure of being worked on by Queen Afua. She was about to apply a healing agent to my body when right before application the congestion in my chest began to break up and disperse. This was quite an extraordinary experience, I might add.

Prepare yourself, for this is no ordinary book. You have in your hand excerpts from a journey to "holiness." The light that channels through the author onto the following pages is a love offering to your health. Read and Be Well.

Dianna Pharr

Foreword

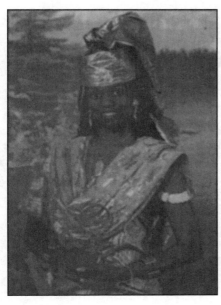

I'VE DEVELOPED the Heal Thyself wellness freedom plan and I've fine-tuned this wholistic freedom plan for over 30 years, day in and day out, season through season, in my waking hours and in my sleep.

This Wellness plan proves that we can indeed heal ourselves from our afflictions and, thus, attain body, mind and spiritual balance. The plan is contained in this text, *Heal Thyself for Health and Longevity.*

The solution to our healing crisis lies in the fundamental question: Are we willing to challenge our appetites, desires and wants? The extent of our change determines whether we are serious about healing ourselves. My years of observation and practice convince me that soul-searching consciousness is the mechanism the Creator has blessed us with to overcome our addictions and our afflictions. We, thus, welcome you to *Heal Thyself for Health and Longevity*, a Path to Purification and Wellness.

Queen Afua

Acknowledgments

MOST HUMBLY, I GIVE THANKS to the Creator for giving me the desire, determination and support to heal myself and for the following people in my life: My mother, Ida, for being my best friend and confidante, and for helping me, along with my two brothers (James and Albert), to raise my children to be whole beings. Ah, my nine aunts, when I see them I get strength. They taught me the power of womanhood.

To my beloved friend and mentor Bob Law, of "Night Talk" (WWRL RADIO), who consistently promotes healing throughout the land, and to his beautiful wife, Muntu, who lovingly propelled me to finish this book.

My most profound love and gratitude to Hru Ankh Ra Semahj Se Ptah, a present-day "King of Kings," for teaching me and so many others the ancient ways of our Khamitic ancestors, and for all those of the Shrine of Ptah, who live and breathe our great and powerful legacy.

Elder Micah, the Godfather of Purification/Natural Healing, inspired me to create my formulas. Many thanks! Love to my sacred editors and literary midwives for diligently assisting in the birth of this work: Carol's faith, Gerianne's unrelenting push, Naikyemi's patience, and Shirley's love.

Love to Queen Esther, for sharing so much of my joy and some of my tears. I'm eternally grateful.

To Lady Prema, sacred songbird and spiritual "auntie," who walked with me faithfully on the Heal Thyself Path of Purification from the early days on and who always makes me mindful of the Creator's presence in my life.

To Cantor Cohen Nabiyim Deborah Yahbah for her divine prophecy about the expansion of my healing work.

To my spiritual reader and long-time friend, Dianna, whose readings have revealed my progress and life's lessons to me in a gentle way.

Much gratitude to my spiritual mother, Empress Akweke, for being the first to inspire me through her extraordinary lifestyle, which led me to be about the "Path of Purification." I give thanks to Empress Ak-weke for honoring me with the title "Queen." Love and Respect.

To my spiritual brother, now an ancestor, Reggie Seagars, who put a healing song in my heart.

To Kalid Nadi, who shared the sounds of his golden flute with many fasters.

To the former staff of the Heal Thyself Center, the fasters, clients and students of the healing path who believed in themselves and the power of purification.

Healing and blessings to David Torain for "gifting" me with our three children who are my most precious gems.

To Richard Bartee, a gracious thank you for your continued support of the healing work.

Blessings to Benyamin for acting as co-Director of Heal Thyself from 1984 to early 1988.

To Rev. Philip Valentine for acting as co-Director of Heal Thyself from late 1984 to 1988.

Immeasurable blessings to Imhotep Gary Byrd and Lloyd Strayhorn who supported me on my Natural Living Crusade throughout the years on the airwaves of Radio Station WLIB.

I salute Baba Ishangi, a masterful cultural teacher, world performer, healer and spiritualist who nursed me and thousands to the shores and through the waters to an Afrikan Beauty, Necessity and Reality.

Much appreciation to Natresha, the Heal Thyself colonic therapist, for purifying the many clients who frequent our center. Tua Ntr for Snt Pa-Ur, and Ingani Choice for teaching and upholding the Heal Thyself Fasting Program over the years. I appreciate your dedication.

Blessings to Hati Ast, a "Divine Mother," whose love is as deep as life itself. To Mzuri, for allowing me to be silent, and for taking me (that winter's night) to the crossroads of my life when I didn't know quite where to turn. To you, a heart-felt embrace.

Thanks to our mother Rosa Parks for acknowledging my work in *Heal Thyself for Health and Longevity* and inviting me to her book signing.

To Stevie Wonder, a shining light, who kindly allowed me to wrap him in herbs, for accepting my tonics and healing waters, and for capturing my heart with a song on my mama's piano... Love.

Much gratitude to Ben Vereen for absolutely embracing Natural Living and Fasting and, thereby, sharing his wellness with his Broadway family of *Fosse* in a Soul Sweat extravaganza.

Much appreciation to Erykah Badu for traveling with the family to administer a Fasting Shut-In, that was held at Hunter College.

Thanks to precious Michael for gathering some of the dancers and stage crew of *The Lion King* in a Soul Sweat as we healed the night away.

Love and healing to the folks of the artistic world who continue to speak and dance and sing, healing tones to our spirit, and for expressing our deepest feelings in a way that inspires us all to flourish.

To all the Afrikan doctors, nurses and health professionals born in the Americas, the Caribbean, and across the globe, those who strive to heal our people, I offer my respect and adoration.

To all the holistic healers and naturopaths of the Four Directions who contain answers I don't have, I honor you. May the Creator continue to bless and protect you and your work.

To the indigenous Americans who maintain the sacred healing sweat lodges and who continue to perform the Sun Dance. Power and strength to your people.

Eternal gratitude to conscious parents who aid in saving the planet by birthing wholistic, organic babies into our world.

Finally, to all those seeking to be healthy, happy and whole, may you have guidance and protection.

Dedication

I LEARNED FROM MY father that you are never too old to grow and heal. My father became a vegetarian at the age of 81 and, together, we put down his walking cane by following Natural Laws. At the age of 82, his arthritis left him and he jogged down the street. Sometimes at night, while I was reading to my father, he would say, "I'm tired... I'm ready to leave this world now." With my innocence, enthusiasm and love, I would say, "Daddy, you are just a child in the eyes of God and you could live 100 years, like the folks you've read about in the Bible, if you live naturally."

Consequently, Daddy had become my best client and believer in healing. In his dying bed, my father sipped garlic juice I gave him. He touched my pregnant stomach, where my son, Ali, was living, and said, "Helen, did you open the Healing Center yet?"

That was more than 20 years ago. He didn't recollect my name very well, for by that time he was in both worlds and making his transition in a hurry, but he did remember my work and envisioned my destiny.

Every now and again when I don't know where to turn in my business affairs, my Daddy comes from the spiritual world and gives me guidance. I want you to know, Daddy, that I appreciate and enjoy those meetings.

So, to Ephraim Robinson, who believed in and raised me on long talks about Marcus Garvey, Martin Luther King and Malcolm X, who lectured on Black folks owning and operating their own businesses and working together for our salvation, I dedicate this book.

This book is also dedicated to my mother, Ida, who loves and supports my work, and my three children, Daoud, Sherease and Ali, who sacrifice with me in the effort to share the Almighty Creator's Purification Laws.

Introduction

My Path to Purification

AT THE AGE OF 17, I developed chronic asthma and severe hay fever. The road of health ignorance and darkness that I was traveling would have surely led to destruction had I not been rescued and led spiritually to the Path of Purification. I probably would have been living in an iron lung by now, had I survived at all.

There was no known cure for me, according to the medical world. I was allergic to almost everything: grass, dust, fur, perfume, mold, several vegetables and fruits, and eggs—all of my life. In fact, the specialist that I was seeing told my mother that I was allergic to too many things and that I really needed to live in a glass house. Even though I was living on a special diet, I was becoming progressively worse.

How it all began is vivid in my mind. It was the evening of August 10th, 1970 at about 8:35 p.m. I sat with my family at the dinner table to partake a "normal" meal of broiled steak, boiled potatoes with butter, muffins and collard greens. For dessert, I had a slice of cake and a glass of milk. I remember the meal being so heavy that after eating I lost all of my energy and had to go to bed immediately. (I later had to outgrow the bad habit of "eating and sleeping" in order to heal myself.)

Ten minutes into my nap, I awoke gasping for breath. My lung had closed down; my face had begun to swell. I remember hearing myself say, "No air can get in or out." I was petrified; it was a labor to gain another breath. I thought, "I am going to die." I cried out, "Daddy, help me! I can't breathe!"

My father held my hand through the night during the bout of sickness, the first of many attacks to come. The word "attack" was so appropriate for I could feel an attack on my mind, body and spirit. It was a total assault and there was nowhere to run.

I was an asthmatic! Every form of medication was given to me, but nothing helped. I deteriorated. I had to learn to live in a suffering state. This disease consumed my young life. Had not my mother told me I'd be alright and that people did not die any more from asthma, I don't know what would have happened to me then. Of course, she was trying to comfort me, for I found out later that people do die from this respiratory disease. It was my belief in my mama's words that carried me and enabled me to clutch onto life. For when evening attacks came, I remember I clung onto her words of hope for dear life. I felt that was all I had to hold onto. I would repeat in my mind my mother's words that I was going to make it to dawn. "I am going to make it through the night 'cause you said I would, and I believe you, Mama. I have faith in you.'" For me, the closest person to God was Mama, and, thus, Mama always told me the truth—and I believed her truth.

Many a night the asthmatic attack was so severe that I would secretly turn on the night light so as not to disturb the rest of the household, and prop up several pillows against the sofa so I could quietly sleep, sitting up all night, enduring eight hours of pain and tightness in my chest. I would wheeze a lot, sleep a little and pray, as I sat in fear of the next breath being my last. This inner turmoil would go on 'til the crack of dawn, for just as the sun was coming up, so too my breath (life) would return—a quiet miracle. Once again, by the Creator's grace and my faith in my Mama's words, I survived another night.

My deepest disappointment was when my doctor told me that it would be impossible for me to take my scheduled college trip to Afrika. He predicted that I would become very sick due to the grass and trees of my lost-but-not-forgotten Motherland.

I did not yet understand that it had been my American meat-and-potatoes diet that had prevented me from being able to go home to Afrika. I had not made the connection between my diet and my health, so I continued to live in this ignorance and poor health for some time.

Three years went by. During these years, I developed arthritis in my shoulder as well as eczema all over my body. Later, I learned that these problems were a result of bad diet, inner rage, depression and not feeling able to express things I needed to express. When we heal, we must be prepared to heal physically, mentally, emotionally and spiritually. We want complete healing.

One summer, a close friend invited me to a vegetarian retreat where I met the famous, late great Afrikan American Master Herbalist for over 50 years, Dr. John Moore, who later became my spiritual grandfather.

Three days before the retreat, I threw away my medication because I was feeling like a junkie who had to take legal drugs to stay alive. Deep in my soul, I prayed that there was another way.

On my arrival at the retreat site, I saw grass and trees. I had no medication; I panicked. Thirty minutes later, I began to wheeze; my eyes became red and bloodshot; my skin began to itch. I felt trapped. "What am I going to do now?" I thought.

A quiet voice inside of me said, "Eat only lemons, grapefruits, and oranges and drink warm water." I did this for 28 hours, and all of a sudden, mucus was being expelled from everywhere, my eyes, nose and mouth. After about 24 hours of releasing in this way, I was able to breathe normally. My eyes became white; my skin stopped itching, and I was emotionally at peace.

For the remainder of the retreat, I listened ecstatically to Dr. Moore and other lecturers speaking on Natural Healing and Nature Cures. A whole new world opened for me; I realized that with faith, determination and a cleansed body Temple, I could finally be healed.

Today, 30 years later, I remain disease-free. I continue to heal myself daily and joyfully. My healing made me realize with the Creator's grace and blessings, that my people, and others who choose nature, no longer have to suffer, and that freedom, spiritual, physical and emotional, is at hand.

These last 28 years or so, I have been led on a crusade to teach and preach "Liberation Through Purification." I have learned to use every lesson as a blessing. My recovery from my illness gave me the determination to support thousands through their healings. My illness, that turned to a healing, has served as a catalyst for the "resurrection of a people."

I do not claim these writings to be the whole story on healing. The other part is within you, other healers and "would-be" healers. However, the portion I'm led to share comes from my heart. Take this and use it wisely.

Glory be to the One Most High.

One

A Cry for
World Healing

Every nation shall read this book as a guide to natural healing—from the Continents to the Poles.

THIS IS A CALL for planetary healing and purification. A global resurrection is mandatory if we are to continue to thrive on earth.

This is a call to the United Nations, to the communities of the world. This is a call to our leaders—political, spiritual, educational, business and artistic—who have an even greater responsibility to purify, lest the people be led to mass destruction.

We have come into the age when our cleansing is most urgent, right here, right now. According to how we disrespect or respect nature and our body Temples, we will experience total devastation and destruction, or total enlightenment and resurrection. From the global to the personal, there is evidence that the necessity for the purification of the heart, mind and body Temple is at an all-time high.

There is bloodshed due to wars. There are increased numbers of crimes in the streets. There are homicides and overcrowded jails. There are battered wives and abused children. There are the slow-death addictions and abuses of drugs and alcohol. There are out-and-out suicides. There are the soaring numbers of cancer victims and victims of the

5

AIDS epidemic (plague). There is premature aging, heart attacks, hysterectomies and mastectomies. There are *crib deaths* due to lack of knowledge, and children born with aging dis-eases passed down from possibly toxic parents or extremely polluted environments.

With mental, spiritual and physical breakdowns everywhere, there is no choice but to purify. The rich, poor, young and old must cleanse if we are going to rise above the diseases of the body, mind and soul.

The Earth is expressing her discontent with how humankind has worked against natural laws. Ultimately, we have worked against ourselves. Our impure thoughts and acts of hate, rage, jealousy, depression and despair have led to the production of impure waters, acid rain, drought, devitalized soil and poisonous air. Equally, our bodies are filled with waste, worms and poisons.

Mother Earth warns us with her earthquakes, hurricanes and volcanic eruptions. Through fire and water, she is cleansing herself of all the filth, just as a woman cleans her womb of tumors by the fire of life-giving foods and water cleansings.

All religious and holy people and ancient spiritual masters of days gone by have shown us the truth and the way; that the foundation for liberation is to fast, to pray and to purify. The ancient masters did not eat of the flesh. They were vegetarians. They were clean.

We, too, must now walk in their footsteps. This way of living holds all the keys for peace on earth, for self-realization, success, health and resurrection for the healing of the planet and humankind.

We must cease our internal and external wars with ourselves and with one another. We must seek to live with a fervor and determination to expunge disease, which runs rampant on this planet due to our unnatural life styles, greed and ears deafened to our own inner voices.

Early one morning, the Creator spoke through my inner voice: "Worry not, my children. Man does not control his destiny, I do. Refocus your eyes. Follow my ways, follow my laws and I will set you free!"

In response to my inner voice and in response to the Creator, I offer the following pledge:

> *I, Queen Afua, born Helen Odel Robinson, am reaching back into the beginning of time and drawing the strength, power and dignity of those ancient times and ancient folks. I affirm for my people and all people—right here and now—that our personal, spiritual and physical liberation is through purification. To all I am able to reach, I will share this Freedom call — "Liberation through Purification!"*

My work and this book are efforts to right some of our wrongs, to give us formulas that help us go beyond mere survival in the coming age.

To my human family, I say: Put the plate down, my sisters and brothers, my mothers and fathers. Let us fast and pray our way out of bondage and darkness into truth and light. Be victorious—for our lives, our souls, our children's children's lives and souls depend upon our purification. Glory be to the One Who Rules the Heavens and the Earth. It was true then as it is true now: *Physical, Mental and Spiritual Liberation Comes Through Purification.*

Let us liberate ourselves from disease and spiritual unrest. Peace can exist on earth, but it must begin with you. From you comes family healing, then community healing, national healing, and finally, global healing.

We must use the Creator's tools to heal ourselves. The tools are fasting, prayer, using herbs, juices, live, sun-ripened foods, hydrotherapy and aromatherapy. We must maintain high and clean thoughts and allow divine, righteous love to flow through every cell so that we may build body Temples of light.

Only the light beings will make it through; only the "shining" ones. There are a chosen few. Are you one of them?

Wake up and rise into a Natural, Divine Way of Living—*Heal Thyself.*

HOW YOU CAN BENEFIT FROM
THE HEAL THYSELF HOLISTIC HEALTH PLAN?

Who   Benefits

The Athlete
- Develops more stamina and endurance.
- Learns to control breathing and acquire stronger, cleaner lungs.
- Increases concentration and becomes physically more flexible.

The Artist
- Becomes more creative. Increases energy.
- Produces an effective stage presence.
- Increases your natural radiance and beauty.
- Increases vocal range, making it higher and deeper; the voice will be fuller.

The Business Person
- Develops brain power and increases memory.
- Aids movement up the corporate ladder.
- Draws money and positive, successful contracts towards you.

Seekers of Physical Beauty
- Experience weight loss and rid their bodies of cellulite.
- Gain clear skin, devoid of acne and a decrease of wrinkles and lines.
- Remove bags from under the eyes.
- Become poised and relaxed.
- Stimulate hair growth.
- Remove body odors.
- Acquire a pleasant speaking tone.

Lovers and Mates
- Experience greater sexual fulfillment, and more intense orgasms.
- Become more loving, gentle and in tune with their inner selves and with their mates.
- Acquire spiritual awareness during lovemaking.
- Have the ability to experience lovemaking as a sacred, divine gift.
- Develop a body that will taste delicious.

Note: Watch with whom you make love. Be sure that he or she cleanses for "we are what we eat."

Who	**Benefits**
The Family	• Shares in a healthy, progressive, strong and loving family unit.
Parents-to-be	*Cleanse for three months to a year before you try to conceive.*
	• You will create a genius child, a love child, a disease-free baby. Many children are born today with cancer, retardation, arthritis, etc. Deep cleansing and rejuvenation before conception may prevent the occurrence of these illnesses.
Parents: Mothers and Fathers	
	• Increase levels of patience.
Elders	• Have fewer/less severe aches and pains.
	• Experience a decrease in tendency toward senility.
	• Have increased energy.
	• Experience a reversal of the aging process and an increase in physical power and strength.
	• Decrease the need for medications.
	• Gain knowledge that life is not over; it's just beginning.
Spiritual Life	• Your prayer life will increase effortlessly.
	• Temptations in the form of drugs or alcohol will be removed from you.
	• You will experience peacefulness and a greater capacity to have divine love.
	• You will have a closer relationship with the Creator.
	• Your "third" eye (spiritual center) will open.

Two

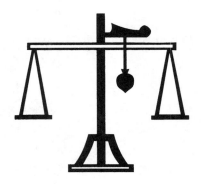

Let the Healing Begin

'Sick and tired of being sick and tired,' then it's time to make a positive stance and begin to journey on the road to wholistic wellness; to unleash your blessings and allow them to flow out freely, from you to others.

As I STAND ON the island of Jamaica looking out on the Caribbean Sea, I speak through my moving meditation. The curtain of the world opens and there are drums and shekeres being played in the background of the heavens. There is gospel music playing. 'Hail to the Most High' is spoken.

I come out on the stage of life and say, "I've come to share with you a gift of healing, not simply because I'd like to, but because I have to—not because I want to, but because I need to."

You see, contained in this Urn (book) is gold dust, a magical gold that is within us. Whenever we are ready to heal, the gold dust becomes activated. The Creator has given us this inner gold by which to "Heal Ourselves." Once that inner gold becomes ignited and begins to shine, we become blissfully at peace and at one.

The healing begins to swell up within me and then I've got to share the feeling, because it's busting out of my toes and running through my fingers and pouring out of my eyes and exploding through my mind.

I've got to share this healing. My gold moves me to share this goodness. I've become so ecstatic about what the Creator has given us so magnificently through air, fire, water and earth that my joy has to be expressed through dancing about. But, that isn't enough.

I have to sing about the healing and still that just isn't enough. Finally, I have to testify about my healing. So I jump for joy, get happy and shout. It has gotten so that I find myself thanking the Creator in every language. Hail to the Most High, Jah, Allah the Most Merciful, Jehovah, Olódùmarè, and Jesus because the healing is so full, so good, so massive it encompasses the world.

Oh, I've been delivered. I feel golden, just like the sun—always vibrating, radiating, glowing and sharing its light. That's why I've got to share my healing. I can't help myself. I love you too much not to share this good feeling.

In this magical Urn is all the gold that's inside of me. I'm going to sprinkle you down and God's going to lift you up. Ralph Carter! Lady Prema! Queen Esther! My Mama! My Daddy in the spirit world! And all my loves! Let the healing begin!

Many years have gone by, sixteen years or more, and I've journeyed through the drama of our healing. I have talked to the elders about the healing, and taught the children about the healing. I've dried thousands of tears of women growing into their healing. I've massaged breast-feeding mothers, given counsel to the brothers, and delivered beautiful babies. I loved my man through his healing. I've been through it all.

It seems the more I've gone through, the more I'm feeling life, feeling free, feeling wonderful simply just to be. By way of my journey, I've purified myself so much until my third eye done opened. I'm getting a vision. I can see the world dancing, and healing, and shouting for joy. Fasters! Healers! Would-be Healers! There's a world healing going on. In all four corners of this earth, there is a world healing going on, in the North, South, East, and West.

As I spread my hands throughout this universe in spirit, body, mind, and soul, I see in my inner vision a world healing going on. All war and destruction has ended. The mama within me and the father within me and within us have said, 'There's a world healing going on.' And so it is. Right now, as we affirm together our healing, may the curtain stay open within your life and may the light of the Creator shine upon you and give you peace. For as sure as the sun sets and the moon rises, know that 'there's a world healing going on.' It's going on within me, within you and within us. So, let the healing begin!

Three

Prepare
Yourself
and Your Home

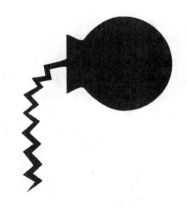

Forgiveness and Thanksgiving are the Keys to Spiritual Preparation for Healing.

AS A SPIRITUAL preparation to embark upon the path of natural living and purification, we must be in a state of constant forgiveness so that we may be forgiven for the sins we have imposed upon ourselves and others. So, let us affirm together: 'Today I forgive all the people, conditions and circumstances that ever hurt me in this life and past lives. For in my forgiving, I begin the process of complete healing. The sickness within me is no more. Instead of holding onto anger, bitterness or sadness, I offer it all up to the Most High.'

We must be in a state of thanksgiving for our many gifts and blessings. Let us give thanks and praise together: 'I spread my arms to the north and south, and my heart to the east and west. I give full thanks and most gracious gratitude for my ancestors who laid the foundation for me to grow, to learn and to reach each beyond the stars. Thank you for showing me the way through the forest and trees. Thank you for being there in spirit. May I walk in your footsteps. May I one day become a wonderful and deserving ancestor.'

To our parents who were the avenues of our arrival to this earth: 'I love you, Mama and Baba (father). You gave me all you had to give and I give thanks. How much of my life can I give you in return?'

To our mates, past and present: 'You taught me my lessons of humanity, how to say "yes" and when to say "no." You taught me the many levels of loving, the many levels of living and the many joys of forgiving.'

To our children and the children of the world: 'You have shown me how to love unconditionally, even when it was painful. Through my pain, I had my greatest births, deepest understanding, and my most intense transformation. Glory, glory, glory.'

'For the bird that passed my window, the butterfly that has landed on my shoulder, the rain that falls and the sun that rises, I give thanks and gratitude to the Creator and to nature. Thank you for providing me with my healing continuously, freely, abundantly and lovingly. I give thanks in my hours of darkness and I give thanks in the light for each divine lesson given to me.

'I give thanks for each additional breath that I am given from the one who rules the Heavens and the Earth, my Great and Divine Mother Father. I give thanks for my life, for giving and sharing life. I give thanks as I ecstatically look forward to all of life's challenges with joy and great expectation.

'Hail to the Most High for forgiveness and thanks-giving. Today, I bear witness to my complete healing. Forgiveness and thanksgiving flow through me. All of my sins are washed away.'

Preparing the Home for Self-Healing

Your home is a reflection of who and what you are and the levels that you've reached in self-awareness. If your house is in order, your personal temple is usually at peace. On the other hand, if your home is out of order, there is usually some internal confusion or unrest within yourself.

Let's use this time not only to cleanse our inner temples but also to cleanse our outer temples. When you come in from the world and enter into your home, allow your home to be a sacred place, a place of refuge, and a place where you can recharge, and gain balance and peace. Let it become a place to prepare you for your work in the world.

Clean out the old to make room for the new. Work within seven-day cycles. Wash all floors. Use Florida water, ammonia, peppermint liquid soap. *Note*: One-teaspoon cinnamon in the cleaning solution brings sweetness to your home.

- If you have an opportunity to paint your home or prayer room, then paint it.

- Clean out closets and drawers. They represent areas of your subconscious, your deepest, most hidden feelings, which must be "cleaned out."

- Throw out all clothing and shoes, which have only been gathering dust.

- Wash and press all clothing in an orderly fashion so that your mornings run smoothly and effortlessly. No last-minute pressing clothes or looking for shoes. That's no way to go into work. If you leave your house scattered, you will find its reflection in the world.

- Open all windows in the house daily for a few moments during the winter months. During the summer months, keep the windows open for complete circulation of the air elements. Allow the air to constantly baptize you and lift you up high.

The Entrance To Your Home

Keep a vase full of fresh Lucky Leaves or a cactus plant near your doorway. You can also place three lemons over the doorway, which you can change periodically. This is Dr. John Moore's spiritual formula to protect your home.

These natural elements spiritually aid in absorbing any adverse forces that are entering your home or even better, will repel them from coming into your sacred space. If you become very pure and holy, then adverse forces will not enter or direct themselves toward your body Temple or your sacred space. Negatives, as positives, are reflections. The body Temple is the inner reflection and must be kept clean and your home is your outer reflection. It must be kept clean. Your thoughts must be purified for thought is the end result of your inner and outer life made manifest.

Helpful Hints about Colors

For best results, when painting our home or even wearing colors on your body Temple, remember these helpful hints about colors:

White	Purification
Violet/indigo	Spirituality and higher mind
Yellow	Higher mind, divine intelligence
Blue	Peace and tranquility
Green	Healing
Soft Pink	Love
Orange	Stimulation
Red	Energy and Productivity

Your Home As A Healing Space

Living Room

Avoid using the living room for constant video and television activity. Such activity creates dulled senses, slow thinking, and radiation poisoning, in most cases. Instead, use your living room as an opportunity for family communication, meditation, exercise or artistic expression.

Keep plenty of plants in the living room for greater oxygen supply. Additionally, have pillows so you can sit low. The low sitting causes flexibility in the body and humbleness in the spirit.

Your Kitchen as a Healing Laboratory

This area of the home is the foundation of higher health and healing to the entire household. The culinary chemist, whoever she or he may be, holds the physical, mental and spiritual blueprints of the family and future generations. The combination of nature's elements that we call food must be alive to give life, must be balanced to maintain balance within, must not be over-seasoned (which irritates) and above all, they must invigorate rather than stimulate. This room must be in total order. The state of mind is of paramount importance in this laboratory, for the emotional energy you entertain during the preparation of your food is the most important ingredient you contribute to the art. Your resulting formula can heal the household or destroy it.

Cleanse your refrigerator and discard all devitalized foods. Their energies can pollute the nearby foods that have higher and more pure rates of motion, i.e. fresh fruits and vegetables.

The following are further helpful hints to you, as a chemist, on the make-up and maintenance of a powerful culinary laboratory.

Purification Kitchen Laboratory Tools

Juicer: Look for a good juicer to extract the juice from vegetables and fruits. Some juicers are not designed to extract the juice of oranges, grapefruits or lemons so you may have to purchase a citrus juicer or a special attachment for your juicer. A good juicer will 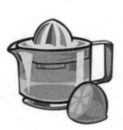 separate the juice from the pulp. You can purchase a juicer at the local health food store or department store. If you can afford to do so, invest in a good one, such as Acme or Champion. The less expensive Oster vegetable and fruit juicer, which can be found in your local department store, is also suggested.

Blender: You can use a blender for mixing your nutrients in with your vegetable or fruit juices or for making fruit shakes and vegetable cocktails.

Measuring spoons and measuring cup:
Carefully measure your nutrients, the waters for your tonics and the amount of juice you are required to take daily.

Sharp knife:
Use to prepare fruits and vegetables for juicing. It is easier if the fruits and vegetables used are cut up into smaller pieces for juicing. It also is better for your juicer.

Cast iron, stainless steel, clay or glass pots; bamboo steamer:
Avoid using aluminum utensils.

Strainer: A small mesh strainer is good for straining herbs from your health tonics and any excess pulp from your juices.

Garlic press:

>Purchase this only if you are going to use fresh garlic cloves, instead of Kyolic, for your Kidney-Liver Flush. (The formula appears in Chapter 6 in Shut-In formula.)

Cutting board:

>Use this to prepare your fruits and vegetables for juicing.

Mugs and drinking cups:

>Have on hand 8-ounce, 12-ounce and 16-ounce drinking glasses for your juices and 12-ounce mugs for your Kidney-Liver Flush.

Large Mason jar:

>Use this to mix and steep your health tonics overnight.

Stainless steel or glass teakettle:

>For boiling your water for your tonic and Kidney-Liver Flush.

Aloe plant: You may use this if you are a little out of tune, or get cut or burned while preparing the foods or herbs in your kitchen laboratory.

You also may want to put a sign over the doorway of your kitchen saying:

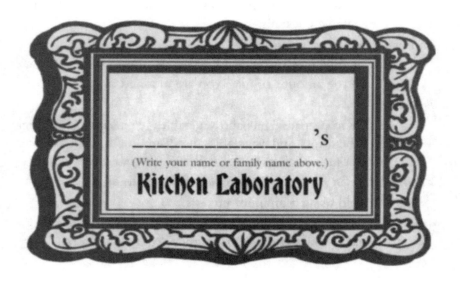

_____'s
(Write your name or family name above.)
Kitchen Laboratory

Water Healing Supplies for your Hydrotherapy Room (Bathroom)

TOOLS	FUNCTIONS
Whirlpool Bath	For circulation, healing and relaxing.
Water Pik	For localized water healing.
Enema bag (qt.)	For purging body Temple.
Squatting stool™	To squat on toilet to allow greater elimination.
Nose rinser:	For deeper, fuller breathing.
(Netipot or Kettle)	
Loofah brush	To cleanse pores of skin.
Small candle	For quiet meditation (when in bath).

For ambiance, add flowers, hanging plants, inspirational posters and sayings to beautify your hydrotherapy room. Make your bathroom beautiful and conducive to relaxation so that it can help you do the work of releasing poisons from your head to your toes. Peace should abound around the toilet, sink, shower, tub and all parts of your hydrotherapy room.

Toiletries

Oatmeal scrub	For soft skin and to remove dead skin.
Natural soaps	Afrikan Black soap, Clay soap, Peppermint soap, etc.
Bath oils	Eucalyptus and Peppermint oils to open your pores for detoxification.
Rosewater	For freshening up.
Almond oil	To soften skin.
Goldenseal Salve	For rejuvenating the skin
Vitamin E oil	For glowing, radiant skin.
Toothpaste	Use Queen Afua's Rejuvenating Clay for teeth and gums or Peppermint and Myrrh toothpaste.

Four

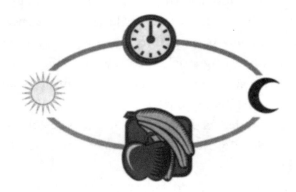

Dietary
Timetable

There is a time, a place, and a season for all, a time for all things; an appropriate time for drinking and eating, a time for personal cleansing, a time for self-rejuvenation, a time to go within and rest from consumption. Get in tune with Divine time and you will be in harmony with self, with the Creator, with nature, with foods and all your relations.

When Should We Eat?

DIETARY TIMETABLE implies that there is a particular time during the day in which we can best handle food. Our body's energy level increases and strengthens as the sun gets stronger in the heavens, and decreases as the sun returns home (*sets*). Our body handles food according to the potency of the sun. If we desire ultimate health and longevity, weight loss and mental clarity, our dietary intake must reflect this in the amounts and kinds of food eaten.

Sunrise

We should eat lightly because we are just coming out of a fast, that is, 4-8 hours of non-eating that we spend sleeping. In the morning, we must not shock the body with heavy foods such as pancakes, meats, fried foods, rolls, etc. or even loud noises. We must gently rejoin body and spirit with a light diet, easy morning movement/exercise and with prayer and meditation. The lighter the sunrise "break-fast," the more in tune we can be spiritually. We will experience a greater energy level and be more mentally alert throughout the day. We should introduce foods into the body Temple that are easier to digest like fruits and fresh juices. For those who are not satisfied with soya or nut milk, one piece of fruit and a cup of herb tea such as chamomile (for the nerves), rosehips (vitamin C) or red zinger (relaxant with vitamin C) will suffice. If the mind is weak in the mornings, take 1 teaspoon of gota kola herb tea with one cup of water, and steep for 30 minutes. For a "morning coffee," that's high in iron, add 3 tablespoons blackstrap molasses to a cup of warm water.

Sun Apex

By midday (lunch-time), the sun is at its strongest point and so are we. Naturally, nutrients will be digested more easily during this time. As a result, we should consume our heaviest meal during this time span. You can use the reminder of the day to exercise as a digestive aid for this midday meal. Such exercise could include walking, or running for the bus, walking up stairs, and reaching and pulling with the arms. Exercise helps the body to quicken its pace in the acts of digestion, assimilation and finally elimination. Your body can have foods such as proteins (soya meats, beans, peas, lentils, baked fish and nuts), complex carbohydrates (starches), steamed vegetables or raw salad. Study the food combination chart (provided later) for greatest digestion of your food. Note that all juices, teas, or water should be taken 30 minutes to 1 hour before or after your meal.

Sun Descent

By late day (dinner time), we are to eat lightly once again; for like the sun, we are to return home and allow the body to become quiet and light again. If we eat after the sun goes down, particularly heavy foods, we will suffer from indigestion, gas, nightmares, bad moods, weight problems and constipation. Food taken beyond the hour of sunset will ferment and poison the system, even when the body is in a resting state.

In the Fall/Winter, your last meal should be taken between 4 p.m. -5 p.m., but no later than 6 p.m., even if you have a late work night. In the Spring/Summer, the last meal should be taken between 7 p.m. -8 p.m. If you must eat after preferable digestion hours, then eat only fruits, fresh vegetables, salads, or drink fresh fruit or vegetable juices.

Within seven days of living according to the Dietary Timetable, you will see a decrease in weight of 4-8 pounds and an increase in morning energy and power. Others will begin to notice that you have a beautiful morning disposition.

To move with the rhythm of the seasons, take note of the following:

Fall/Winter: We eat heavier foods to build heat in our bodies. We also hibernate (*sit in*) more. There is a greater possibility for mental depression, aches and pains, shortness of breath, and colds and fevers. During this season, there is a greater need for meditation, quiet movements and planning for the future (Spring-coming out).

Spring/Summer: We are ready to venture out into the world. We are more active. To keep up with the season, we eat lighter and, naturally, do more fasting. Act upon winter meditations. It is planting time!

To do differently will cause our bodies to rebel by getting sick. Overeating, especially in the summer, causes tiredness, skin eruptions, high blood pressure, edema, etc.

Five

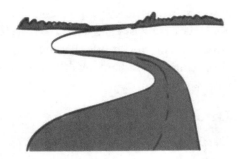

Before
You Begin

It is suggested that you read this entire section before beginning your two-cycle cleansing. It is especially important to read Detoxification and Breaking the Nutritional Fast to avoid or limit a cleansing Crisis.

Hydrotherapy

To restore and to purify oneself with the use of water as a form of natural treatment.

TAKING WARM WATER soaks can help in relaxing your body and your mind. Taking salt baths to draw out negative toxic states, stress, anxiety and bring forth a state of serenity began in the Nile Valley of Smai Tawi in Afraka as a form of natural therapy. These baths were taken as purification rites to help one to prepare for spiritual healing, which aided in healing the body Temple as a whole.

In this age and time, we are able to continue this purification within our homes and our personal temples, by converting our bathrooms into hydrotherapy rooms, by taking 1-4 pounds of Epsom salt or 1 to 2 pounds of Dead Sea salt or hot water soak for 20 to 30 minutes. Begin by lighting a white candle for clarity or a blue candle to symbolize serenity or simply close your eyes and meditate on your inner light, becoming more vibrant as you gently soak your sacred Temple. While soaking in the tub to enhance your cleansing of body, mind, and spirit, drink a pint of lemon water by adding 1 to 2 lemons or limes to your drinking water. While in your bath, perform self-massage from head to toe, and mentally, physically and emotionally give yourself permission to release relationships, situations, environment, and foods that are toxic as you affirm that joy, peace, and abundant and radiant health will flow in and through your life from this day forward.

Detoxification

Detoxification is to release oneself from poison. According to the dictionary, a poison is a substance causing illness or death when eaten, drunk, or absorbed even in relatively small quantities. A poison is something harmful or destructive to happiness or welfare, such as an idea or emotion. Mental, emotional and physical poisons are relationships, environmental or food-related, and can result in fear, anger, hostility, depression, stagnation, high blood pressure, tumors, cancer, respiratory infections, diabetes, arthritis, and related ailments.

You may prevent or eliminate poisonous, destructive habits from your life by embracing the ancient art of purification through internal and external cleansing via enemas, colonics, self-massage, taking baths, establishing a natural living, vegetarian life style and performing seasonal nutritional fasting, affirmations and healing prayers as well as by associating with positive, progressive company.

Detoxification is not a one-time experience. Detoxification is an ongoing aspect of natural living. When one is fully detoxified, one can be dis-ease free, with the ability to experience excellent health, greater longevity and vitality. Through detoxification, one will reverse the aging process and become more youthful—regardless of age.

We have accumulated poisons at conceptions, according to how our parents lived. Their collective poisons (dis-ease) as well as their state of health has been passed on to us through our bloodline.

Through ignorance of nature's health laws, we continue to accumulate poisons throughout our lives until such time as we call on nature to help us purify from our mental, emotional and physical dis-ease.

If one falls off the path of purification and stress and challenges revisit you, and you find yourself backsliding; by all means, carry no guilt. Just start over again; affirm your wellness; get in tune and get back in line. Observe patience and, remember, you did not get sick overnight; it's going to take time and devotion to transform yourself. Self-healing is a life-long process; it's a way of life.

Dare to be Great! Purify more! Once you start fasting (i.e. living off of fruit and vegetable juices), your body will begin to detoxify, getting rid of wastes and poisons that have been in the body for years. All fasters experience cleansing reactions at the onset of their fasts. First of all, don't be alarmed, for it is a natural reaction and is to be expected. You may experience anywhere from one to three different cleansing reactions. The more preparation you put into starting the fast (eating more fruits and vegetables), the fewer experiences of 'faster's detox' you will have. Here's a list of some things you may experience during the first few days of fasting:

Fasting or Cleansing Crises

Aches and Pains	Nightmares	Dizziness
Weakness	Blurred Vision	Heavy Breathing
Tiredness	Vaginal Discharge	Fevers
Skin Eruptions	Mental Confusion	Flatulence (Passing Gas)
No Patience	Depression	High Blood Pressure
Headaches	Mood Swings	Shortness of Breath

These reactions come from a history of poor diet, nighttime eating, too much starch, too much sugar and heavy meat intake, along with consuming excessive fried foods and dairy products. The reactions you experience could last from an hour to 2 or 3 years.

The best way to help your body adjust to these changes is to first discontinue taking all fruit juices until the symptoms subside. Continue to take your vegetables juices; this will stabilize and strengthen the body before deeper cleansing can continue through taking fruit juices. (*Note*: Juice combinations will be given later.)

Take enemas immediately, using only warm water in a quart-size enema bag. Discontinue taking salt baths for two days. Take warm showers instead. Give yourself a vigorous massage starting at your feet and working upwards toward your heart. You may even want to have a professional massage.

Discontinue taking your Kidney-Liver Flush Formula

. Detoxifying the liver and kidneys increases circulation, cleanses the colon and breaks up mucus throughout your system. (The formula appears in Chapter 6.) Replace it with the juice of one lemon, three tablespoons of cold-pressed olive oil and eight ounces of warm water. Also drink a mixture of dandelion and alfalfa tea. *(Use 2 teaspoons of each herb in 2 cups of water. Steep for 2 hours.)* Get more rest and sleep.

If you follow these instructions, your cleansing reactions should be over within one to three days. If the symptoms persist, please contact your fasting consultant or get an emergency colon cleansing. Some fasters who were on a light vegetarian diet before fasting usually found that they did not experience any of the reactions listed.

One key thing to remember throughout fasting is to constantly give yourself intense prayer treatments. Call on your God for your restoration and healing with your heart and soul. If you cleanse and rejuvenate regularly and consistently, you can expect to rid the body of all the diseases that were mentioned earlier, as well as eliminating all other chronic diseases, such as: *High Blood Pressure; Arthritis; Asthma, Hay Fever and Allergies; Female Disorders (cysts, tumors, heavy menstruation); and Prostate Gland Disorders.*

Note: For heavy bleeding, take Shepherd's Purse in the form of a herbal tea, from a basic formula—three teaspoons to three cups of water. Boil your water first; turn off the water, and add your herb. Let it steep for 4 hours or overnight for a more potent formula. Then, strain and drink.

Commonly asked Questions about the Natural Living and Nutritional Fasting Process

1) *How do I get my nutrients (minerals and vitamins) during the fast?*

A: Your nutrients are in the spirulina, herbs and juices you will take.

2) *Will I have enough energy during the fast?*

A: If you eat lightly (fruits, vegetables and water) for 1 week or more before a fast and take at least 1-2 enemas or herbal laxatives, you will be on "high" throughout the fast. If not, increase your spirulina or *Heal Thyself Nutritional Formula* to an additional teaspoon with juice and take an additional enema for greater energy.

3) *Can I go to work while fasting?*

A: By all means! The Urban City Fast, the original name of my Nutritional Fasting Method, is designed to allow you to live as much of a "normal" life as possible. If you prepare 1-2 weeks for your fast, you should have no problems while working. During your work hours, your fasting should be a pleasant experience.

4) *How do I handle social engagements, holidays and eating out at restaurants?*

A: Invite your friends or business associates out to a vegetarian restaurant. Learn the various food alternatives and follow some of the recipes within this book. There are prepared meat substitutes in most health food stores, or you may prefer to prepare your meat alternatives in your own kitchen.

5) *Will I feel deprived?*

A: View your cleansing as a gift that you are giving to yourself, the 'Gift of Life.' See the rejuvenation process as a fun and exciting journey or like the beautiful lotus opening up within you. Follow the 'Food Alternative List' that is within this book. You are not going to be able to eat many of the foods you are used to eating. However, the alternatives are healthier.

6) *What if people make fun of me?*

A: Take the path of least resistance. Laugh with them, then share your tabouli and okra, tofu dip with seaweed crackers, freshly prepared pear juice or banana ice cream. You may have a convert.

7) *Suppose my spouse thinks I'm crazy?*

A: Prepare a natural bubble bath and add rose petals to the water. Put on soft music as you welcome your spouse in a bath fit for a king or queen. Massage your spouse's feet with almond oil. While your spouse is in a tub, serve fresh pressed fruit juice in a long-stemmed glass. Do this just as s/he emerges from the bath. Have a freshly prepared salad, steamed vegetables with a vegetarian protein or baked fish waiting. Put a candle and flowers on a table. Your spouse will no longer think you are crazy. S/he will love the change in you since you started the path of purification and will probably join you on it.

8) *Is it necessary to take a daily enema?*

A: Yes. Your body is releasing toxins daily. An enema will ease the burden that the body is going through in trying to eliminate the waste. Your colon is in a state of rest while you are fasting so you will not be eliminating as much waste on your own. As a result, if poisons that have not loosened are left unattended in the body, the body will feed off its own waste. You will then experience headaches, anger, dizziness, blurred vision, etc. Taking daily enemas will ward off these symptoms.

9) *What is a colonic?*

A: A colonic is a form of hydrotherapy. It is a deep cleansing of the colon. Between 5-15 gallons of water flow in and out (through) your colon carrying out old, impacted waste, gas and toxins.

10) *I experienced a headache during the first several days. Why and what can I do to stop it?*

A: You are experiencing a 'faster's crisis.' Take enemas immediately. Discontinue drinking fruit juices for 24 to 36 hours. To stabilize yourself, drink only vegetable juices. Discontinue the Kidney-Liver Flush. Just drink lemon juice and water for your breakfast. Take only showers during this time. No salt baths. In addition, rest as much as you can.

11) *Why is it important to take Epsom salt baths?*

A: The salt and water is like that of an ocean bath. It helps to relax the body and release stress. It also draws poisons out through the pores.

12) *I felt dizzy while in the bath. Why and what can I do about it?*

A: You are eliminating toxins from poisonous foods and drugs taken into your system. If you feel dizzy, decrease your salt bath from 4 to 2 pounds. By the next bath, try to use 3 to 4 pounds of salt. If your diet has been light, you'll be able to take more salt.

13) *What if I stray?*

A: Don't put yourself down in any way. Love, support and nurture yourself throughout your healing process. It takes time to grow.

Take an enema or herbal laxative, healing bath or vegetable juices immediately. These forms of natural healing will put you back on track and in harmony with yourself. The more you actively do the correct things the less likely you are to stray.

14) *How do you know when you are ready to go to the next level?*

A: You will no longer crave particular foods. That is, you will begin to eat fewer foods and desire more fresh juices and more salads. The more you cleanse, take enemas, herbal laxatives, drink vegetable juices, the less you will desire heavy foods.

15. *Should I discontinue taking my medication when I begin your fast or any other?*

A: Do not discontinue taking your medication without your doctor's consent. As you use natural foods, herbs and juices to rejuvenate your body, your doctor will see an improvement in your health and lessen the quantity of medication or will even remove you from it altogether. Have patience. Returning your system back to a state of total health takes time.

Some of these questions were formulated by my friend, lawyer, devotee of purification and author of *The Heal Thyself Natural Living Cookbook*, Dianne Ciccone, and Marcia Lily, a devotee of purification for over nine years. I thank them dearly for being in tune with the heartbeat of the people, knowing what questions needed answering.

Six

Fasting and Cleansing for a Glorious Life

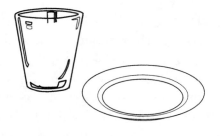

I want to open you up to heaven within, by welcoming you to the Heal Thyself Path of Purification. As you travel on this Wellness journey, expect to release pounds of emotional and physical toxins from your body Temple. The goal is 100 percent wellness in the Body, Mind and Spirit to develop a body free of disease. In the spirit of transformation, your body Temple will gain inner and outer beauty, housed within a loving disposition. Spiritually, you will advance on your journey. Joy and peace will radiate from your being. Expect Your Inner Light to shine ever so brightly in every phase of your new existence.

What is Fasting?

THERE ARE VARIOUS types of fasts, such as the water fast, fruit juice fast, wheatgrass fast, etc. The religious (spiritual) fast is the original fast. During a religious fast, only water is taken into the body. In a "dry" religious fast, the food and drink is totally that of "the spirit."

In nature, when an animal is sick, it will fast until it is well, or it will eat only green grasses of the fields. When we, humans, are in harmony with ourselves, we also know to fast if we become unbalanced and need healing, or if we desire greater spiritual direction.

Sometimes when we become ill, we eat crackers and chicken soup. Unfortunately, this is not a healing thing to do. At this time, we should use a nutritional fasting method to heal and cleanse the body of poisons that have accumulated from eating meats, starches, sugar, cooked oils, and junk food. Sickness is the body's way of rebelling against disrespect and pollution.

There also has been disrespect for our environment. As a result, the air we need to breathe and our waters are polluted. The earth that grows our food has been devitalized. Due to our disrespect of nature, the very elements we need for healing are in crisis, especially in the urban areas. We can no longer only drink water for survival, as did the ancients. Even if we went to more rural areas in order to fast, we would experience violent, detoxification crises due to our years of inner body pollution and dietary ignorance.

I have developed a nutritional fasting method that will cleanse the body Temple with little or no stress. I recommend freshly pressed fruit juices and purified or distilled water to purify, rejuvenate and strengthen the body. I also recommend specific vegetable juices as well as herbs (spirulina and wheatgrass), enemas, herbal laxatives and colonics. Healing baths and exercise also are major components of this fasting method. The body is fed all the necessary vitamins and nutrients. As a result, the oftentimes, uncomfortable, cleansing reactions are lessened, and you are able to maintain sufficient balance while both cleansing and leading your everyday life (family and home care, away-from-home occupations, study and school, etc.) You will experience emotional balance (unlike when on a strict water fast when you might experience mood swings or nightmares). The chlorophyll and vegetable juices aid in emotional harmony and physical strength. The fruit juices detoxify your various organs gently and lovingly.

Chlorophyll is encased in green plants that grow from the soil on land or in the sea. Chorophyllis (plants) are charged by the sun, which provides energy for plants to photosynthesize the materials necessary for human growth, i.e. carbohydrates, proteins and fats. Chlorophyll detoxes and rejuvenates tissues, cells, blood, arteries and nerves.

The more that we consume chlorophyll, in form of eating green leaves like salad and herbs as well as green vegetable juices and wheatgrass, the healthier our skin, hair and bones, the purer our thoughts, and the more harmonious and healthy our relationships past, present, and future will be. Chlorophyll consumption brings heaven on earth within and without. I would go so far as to say that if a community, a country, or even the world consumes chlorophyll consistently (1-2 times a day): we would see an end to world famine, dis-ease and war.

Fasting... Who? Why?

Renew yourselves and fast, for I tell you truly, that Satan and his plagues may only be cast out by fasting and by prayer. Go by yourself and fast alone and show your fasting to no man. The living God shall see it and great shall be your reward. Fast 'til Beelzebub and all his evil depart from you and all the angels of our Earthly Mother come and serve you. For I tell you truly, accept fasting, or you shall never be freed from the power of Satan and from all diseases that come from Satan. Fast and pray fervently, seeking the power of the Living God for your healing.[1]

By fasting you will call back the Lord of your body and the angels. ... Each day that you continue to fast and pray, God's angels blot out each year of your evil deed from the books of your body and your spirit and when the last page is also blotted out and cleansed from all your sins, you stand before the face of the Creator pure and whole.[2]

After fasting, the body has purged the blood of toxins, clogging waste and decaying and diseased cells, then healthy cells are built of better material to replace those cast out of the body during the fast. That is regeneration. That is the Secret of the Ancient Masters. Know the law and observe it. That is the way to keep your body vigorous.

In ancient days, man ate only the green live foods and fruits of nature and drank pure water. They ate less in a day, perhaps, than modern man eats in one meal. The duration of their youth extended

---

[1] Szekely, Edmund Bordeaux, ed. and trans. *The Essene Gospel of Peace* Book 1. International Biogenic Society, 1981.

[2] Ibid, pg. 29

over several centuries (Gen. 5:32), and they lived almost a thousand years.

The ancient masters recognized fasting as the great remedial measure and resorted to it in instances of illness. Fasting twice in the week was a common custom in the days of Jesus. The disciples of John fasted often. David fasted 40 days. Jesus fasted 40 days. Gandhi fasted to get the British out of India. These wise men knew how to promote health and prolong life and free themselves from bondage of any and all kinds.

Each day that you continue to fast and pray, God's angels blot out one year of your evil deeds from the book of your body and cleansed from all your sins, you stand before the face of God. (Essene Gospel of Peace, Vol. 1, p. 29) You must fast one day for each year that you've lived to totally purify yourself. Example: If you are 32-years-old, then you should fast for 32 days. If you are 26, then fast for 26 days and so on. Once you enter the kingdom of God through fasting, you receive prosperity, divine love, health, happiness and peace.

Purification for Spiritual and Physical Liberation

The one thing that all the religions have in common is 'fasting and praying.' This fasting and praying is to bring about liberation on every front. We, as a people, are governed by divine law. The highest law is fasting and prayer. If this is done diligently by the planetary members, the planet could function on a higher frequency and bring an end to pain and suffering.

Peace and harmony can occur on Earth, but, in order for this to occur, we all must in our various religions and walks of life strengthen, double and quadruple our efforts at fasting. Fasting must come to be a way of life. We should proceed with physical and spiritual haste due to the alarming conditions afflicting the planet at this time.

Moslem fast:

During the holy month of Ramadan, Moslems fast for 40 days. During this time, they neither drink nor eat anything between sunrise and sunset.

Christian fast:

On every Friday during Lent and on Good Friday, Christians don't eat or drink. Christians uphold the teachings of Moses, Elijah, and Jesus (Yeshua), who fasted for 40 days and 40 nights. Daniel fasted for 21 days and also was a strict vegetarian. Blessings to Elder Micah, for this information.

Fast of Jews/Israelites:

They fast on a "Day of Atonement" once a year for repentance. The ancient Israelites ate only manna (a sea vegetable like spirulina/an algae from the ocean) for 40 years. They were not allowed to eat any meat.

Fast of Hare Krishnas:

The fast of Kadasi is done twice a month. For 24 hours, one goes without water or sleep. One remains in a state of constant prayer and chanting. This is for the purpose of greater spiritual awareness and to be given more time to glorify God and to transcend the bodily demands. There are three other levels to their fast that are less intense. Blessing to Hla Dini Shakti, a devotee of Hare Krishna.

Fast of Indigenous Americans:

This fast is done during general ceremonies, vision quests and the sun dance for the purpose of purification and healing. The fasting process varies from nation to nation. Blessings to Oscar Moreno, an indigenous American sweat lodge leader, for this information.

Yoruba Religious Fast

The New Year is a time for fasting. Fasting varies according to the faster's position in the community and what he/she is trying to achieve. Priests have the responsibility to foresee what must happen for the new period, so they go through a period of purification to be able to receive the holy messages. When they have achieved this period of "sacrifice," they become lighter and one with the Divine spirit.

Most initiations have a period of fasting. The older you are, the longer you fast. Fasting is not only looked upon as a cleansing, but as a discipline, particularly for spiritualists who have to work long hours communing with the spirits. In various practices, it is a way to show the Divine in one's self, to remove one's self from the worldly pursuits.

Normally, during this kind of fasting a person withdraws and does a total fast, which means no social activity and no sexual intercourse. The person does take liquids and may only come out to take part in rituals. Everyone participating in the rituals looks to those who have been in seclusion for the divine wisdom that comes as a result of their sacrifices. During the withdrawal period, the person is not just fasting, but praying and performing rituals. Often, there are periods of chanting and singing. The person stays within an incubation state during which he/she hopes to receive the divine message.

Sometimes, an 'adept' person will be allowed to come into the sacred area to record what the person might say in this trance-like state. Once the person awakes, the 'adept' person will inform him/her of everything that happened. The 'adept' person must be very wise because it is not only words for which they are listening. The prostrate body itself may get up and dance in a trance state, and languages may come from the mouth that the 'adept' person has not heard.

The 'adept' person also is in a state of fasting, but has himself or herself on a more elementary level and has not secluded himself or herself as the other person has done. The reason for this is because the adept does not want to be charged up by the spiritual world and rendered unable to record the information from the one who is in the trance-like state. Baba Ishangi, Yoruba Priest.

Make fasting a way of life regardless of your own particular spiritual and/or cultural affiliation. Help to actualize miracles on earth.

Fasting Success Chart

Purification is the Key to Success.
The Benefits of Fasting and Cleansing are Unlimited.
Set your Sights High as you Purify into Victory.

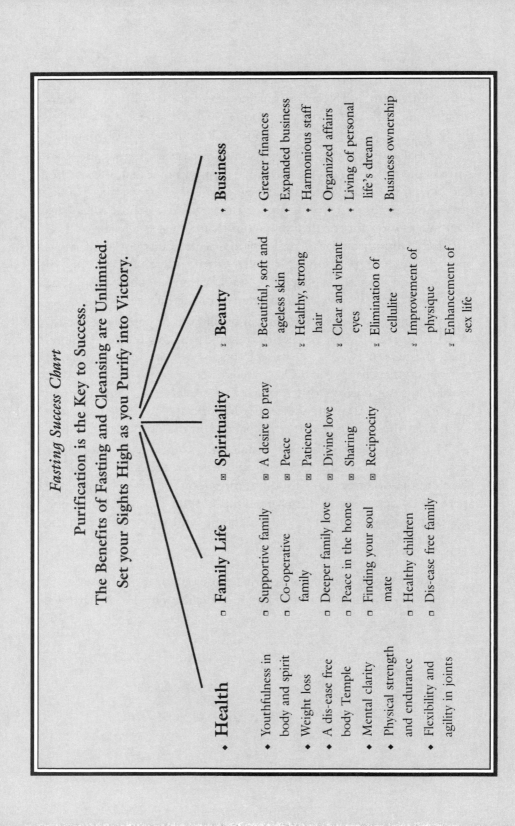

- **Health**
  - Youthfulness in body and spirit
  - Weight loss
  - A dis-ease free body Temple
  - Mental clarity
  - Physical strength and endurance
  - Flexibility and agility in joints

- **Family Life**
  - Supportive family
  - Co-operative family
  - Deeper family love
  - Peace in the home
  - Finding your soul mate
  - Healthy children
  - Dis-ease free family

- **Spirituality**
  - A desire to pray
  - Peace
  - Patience
  - Divine love
  - Sharing
  - Reciprocity

- **Beauty**
  - Beautiful, soft and ageless skin
  - Healthy, strong hair
  - Clear and vibrant eyes
  - Elimination of cellulite
  - Improvement of physique
  - Enhancement of sex life

- **Business**
  - Greater finances
  - Expanded business
  - Harmonious staff
  - Organized affairs
  - Living of personal life's dream
  - Business ownership

When and Why to Fast

During your birthday month:

> In this month, you will be receiving many messages on how to live out the coming year. Keep in mind that you are the ultimate spiritual reader of your own life. No one will know you better than you yourself and Almighty God the Creator. Fast and pray for all doors to open physically and spiritually.

Fast on your Holy day:

> Fast 24 hours every week on your 'Holy day' or 'Accra Day,' which is the day of the week on which you were born.

Fast every seasonal change:

> To welcome in each season, fast 3, 7, or 21 days. If you fast before each season, you will prevent getting any of the illnesses that particular season brings. Fasting helps prevent your body from being off balance. This is especially true during the spring season. If we fast right before and up until the first of spring, we will be showered with abundance, health, wealth, joy and inner peace. Spring also is a good time to begin new projects. Cleansing during this time will assure success in the project. Spring is the time for renewal, cleansing, beauty and coming out. Be in tune and receive your divine gifts.

During menstruation:

> Women should fast two days before the onset of their menstrual flow and all during their menstruation to prevent or minimize pre-menstrual syndrome (PMS), headaches, pain, heavy bleeding and clotting, mood swings and nausea.

Fast to unblock/to clear the way:

> If you are experiencing blockages in your life in the form of lack of money flow, in relationships, on your job, in your profession, in your heart or your health, then fast and purify to clear any lack or limitation.

The How of the 21-Day Nutritional Fast

Queen Afua is the originator of the 21-Day Urban City Group Fast and the 21-Day New Year's Fast. Her fasting method has been used by several other centers throughout the New York metropolitan area.

For advanced students of fasting, the 21-Day Fast is very effective, particularly if done as the seasons change or to effect major changes in your life quickly. This is what you can expect for each week of your 21 days.

Week One: (**Degree 1**, 1–7 days): Elimination of old waste, a rapid clearing within the physical body. This week is when you must pull on your strength to get through the first 3-4 days of fasting. These days —separate the weak from the strong. If you pass these days, you have pretty much eliminated problems thereafter. The "faster's crisis" usually occurs during the first 3-4 days. Follow the instructions included in this book to come out of a crisis as quickly as possible.

Week Two: (**Degree 2**, 8–14 days): This week you become physically stronger—more than ever before. You have more endurance; your body becomes more flexible because the poisons are coming out of the joints. You are able to do things with your body Temple that you did 5-10 years ago. You can walk faster, and have fewer problems walking up stairs. Your breathing will be deeper and fuller. Your mind will be sharper and more crea-tive. Your skin will glow. That book or proposal that you were trying to write previously is now being written effortlessly. We think we might have less energy when we fast. If you use this method of cleansing and rejuvenating, you will have more energy with each given day that you fast.

Week Three: (**Degree 3**, 15–21 days): This is the week when you open up spiritually, when you can hear that still, small voice of NTR, Most High Allah, Almighty God. You are now in your divine state, like that of a holy wo/man. You are more peaceful, relaxed, slow to anger, if at all, more tolerant of others, stress-less and joyous. You smile and laugh more now and you can see the beauty of life. Others will look up to you and ask guidance in their affairs for the light of wisdom, spiritual beauty and peace is flowing through you. Your aches and pains are gone physically, spiritually and emotionally. Repeat the 21 days often if you desire to maintain a high state in an impure world. Fasting is a way for you to truly become "high." Taking drugs and alcohol is not getting you high, it's taking you low. If we all fasted throughout the world, crime, violence and war would be eliminated on the planet Earth.

Once you come off a long fast, eat only fruits and vegetables for 14 days. If you come off the fast and begin eating even whole grains and vegetable proteins or meat, you will reverse the benefits of the fast and get sick. So, eat light foods, continue drinking your juices and stay in peacefulness.

Alternating the Nutritional Fasting and Natural Living method of diet is an excellent life style. It provides for body cleansing with little or no residual stress or strain. You can fast and rejuvenate in this manner without supervision.

When embarking on the 21-Day Fasting Program, it is advised that you seek supervision from a knowledgeable person experienced in guiding you through this longer fasting process.

With each fast you do, you are constantly spiraling up the pyramid toward the top of consciousness, never to return to the land of darkness. You are constantly moving toward more light, brilliance, clarity, power and peace.

Talk Fast

For a period of time daily for spiritual strengthening, particularly during a fast, one should avoid talking for 1-2 hours. This is called your hour of power. This process develops meditation opportunities. Once you peacefully close the portals called the lips, the other portals of communication become more activated, such as the "third eye" and crown chakras. From these centers, you are able to "hear" the Holy Spirit talk through and to you. When these chakras are open, you receive inner spiritual guidance in your daily affairs. This exercise also helps to detoxify your thoughts and release adverse thought processes. It then allows for your mind to experience higher thoughts and visions.

Fasting For World Peace and Health

No more internal or external wars;
there is hope, but we must fast and pray.

Families:

Guide your family members to do consistent fasting together and watch the love build in the family unit.

Teachers:

Take your students through a 3-7 day fast or live food diet weekly. Watch the improvement in your students' performance.

PTA Members:

Fast for 2 days before each meeting and see how smoothly the meeting goes and how much work is accomplished.

CEOs: Have your company members fasted from 24 hours to 3-7 days monthly? If so, have you observed that less sick leave time is taken, that there is greater cooperation among your staff, and that sales have increased. Employees will be happier on the job because the atmosphere will be so pleasant. Fasting is cost effective for the company. Hire a fasting expert to motivate and guide your staff weekly and monthly.

Unions: Ms. Anna Mae Massey, Chairwoman of the Health Committee under the leadership of Mr. Al Diop, President of the largest municipal labor union #1549 DC 37, as a keynote speaker, was able to inform and inspire approximately 200 union members of the value of fasting and cleansing. These union members went on a weekend health retreat. They ate light, healthy foods, drank fresh juices, received healing massages and attended workshops on stress management, holistic health, nutrition, food alternatives and exercise. The participants felt love and gave love that weekend. More unions and businesses need to follow this format.

Presidents, National and Civic Leaders:

You should fast every seasonal change for 7-21 days and 24 hours weekly. Decisions made for a country would become the highest decision for the greater good. A president should encourage citizens to fast 24 hours weekly or 1 to 3 days a month for unity and purity. They should fast to fight crime and bring peace throughout the land. Gandhi fasted to give his people freedom. When the people are pure, there is peace. The violence, in the cities and in the land, is greatly due to "fast foods" (causing fast death). High sugar intake is causing over-reaction, hyperactivity and mental depression. Eating meat causes people to become more violent and animalistic in nature.

Heads of State:

Prior to convening the General Assembly of the United Nations, the representatives should fast for 3 days. This would help prepare them for their tasks of holding peace talks and making decisions that affect the world.

Ministers, Imams, Priests, Rabbis and all Religious Leaders:

You should fast 1-3 days weekly or 7 days a month to live totally on the Holy Word and to be a living example of purity in body, mind and spirit. The cleansing of the leaders will increase the number of followers on particular spiritual paths. There will be more light, love and wisdom coming from the spiritual leader when s/he is living as the ancients by: "fasting and prayer." Spiritual leaders should encourage their congregations to fast on holy days, to eat only spiritual food on those days (not the food of the earth) so that, before and after the service they will be living and breathing the Spirit. Also, if consistent fasting is encouraged, there will be little or no sickness among the followers. With no more high blood pressure, weight problems, asthma, or premature aging, the members will receive healing spiritually and physically by the example of their leaders' guidance and life styles. "Be ye perfect" and purified.

Purification and Rejuvenation as a Way of Life

A wonderful, fantastic, ecstatic, fulfilling way of living. A gift supreme. Explosive! Oh, so powerful! Makes you feel clean on the inside. Look beautiful on the outside. Embrace your healing, digest it, caress it, fall back on it, move forward with it, stand on it, lean on it, and rest on it. It will build you into a perfect temple of pure light, love, wealth and health.

Combining the Nutritional Fasting and Natural Living programs harmonizes the body, mind and spirit. The body, mind and spirit grow and develop collectively and in unison. As you rise and graduate to higher levels in your fasting and natural living, you will bear witness to your heightened spiritual and mental progression. As you work through these various levels, observe how fear, anger, depression, anxiety, and lack of faith fall from you. Observe instead that with each step of purification you advance toward perfection. Observe how a greater capacity for love, how peace, faith, humility, wealth and health radiate through, around and about you.

On the mind:

The Creator will live in your mind and thoughts. You will gain greater intelligence, and creativity that is boundless and unlimited.

On physical wealth:

You will become more prosperous. Our Mother/Father God has many mansions. Because you are the sons and daughters of a great Creator, you are the heirs and heiresses to the throne. If you will but allow the Divine Holy Spirit to guide you and keep you in your business affairs, you shall be triumphant. As you move with joy and great expectation through these high degrees of purification and rejuvenation, your whole world opens like that of a thousand-petal lotus. All is contained in the crown chakra of your being. Once purified, your centers can be activated and you can become pure light and love. As you continue to cleanse your body Temple, that still, quiet, inner voice is able to guide you so that you may be victorious in all your affairs. So, go on and grow through freshman, sophomore, junior and senior levels. Become like Methuselah, who lived to be 976 years of age, and the other ancients who lived for hundreds of years because they were in harmony in body, mind and spirit.

Preparation for Prayer
such as the Heal Thyself Purification Prayer

The Prayer you are about to utter should be spoken upon the rising of the sun, after one has taken a healing bath or shower and has brushed one's teeth and massaged gums with the Rejuvenation Clay. If you are on a special fasting and cleansing program, put on a white robe or wrap a white cloth around your body Temple to signify purity and then anoint yourself with sage or frankincense and myrrh oil.

Now, let us pray, meditate and give thanks, for no matter what has happened in the past, this is a new day and this is your time for healing yourself. Be blessed.

Heal Thyself Purification Prayer

Mother/Father, Creator of the Heavens and of the Earth, make us a New People, New Flesh and Bones, Blood and Veins, Hearts and Minds, a Revitalized People, Spirit full of love and grace. Give us the strength, endurance and faith to live, as you would have us live, a clean life, a purified life; a natural and wholesome life.

Mother/Father Creator, I come pure so that I may be worthy of your blessing of everlasting peace, love, power, joy and radiant health.

Right now, touch my heart, my mind and my soul so that I may walk, talk, think, do and feed my body Temple clean foods.

I give thanks and praise to the Creator for absolute healing rests in your eternal hands, and only through your working, through me, can I heal myself.

Upon the dawn of each day, by way of my purification, I commit and devote myself to you, Creator. Discipline, Natural Living and Determination in the way of purification will carry me through. No more death, destruction and dis-ease. This is true for cleanliness is Truth, Light and Divine Grace.

Dearest Creator, I am willing to be, as you would have me be, a shining example of purity in word, thought and deed.

Dearest Creator, remove the wickedness, the wars, the violence on this Earth that flesh-eating brings. Purify me of the desire for any poisonous ways that plague this Earth.

As I stand before you in prayer, Holy Spirit about you and all within and around you, I call on your Angels (Neteru) of Air, Fire, Water, Earth, to remove all temptation from my path and grant me the power not to stray nor sway to the left nor right, but to stay on the Royal Road of Purification.

You've lifted me up and moved me through so that I may be a cleansing champion of your light.

In our pure, natural state, Mother/Father Creator of the Heavens and of the Earth, you made us; you made us well and full of light, so it is to you, I give thanks and praise; as I commit myself daily to live in a righteous and pure way.

Heal Thyself 365-Day Road Map to the Path of Purification

What you are witnessing on this road map is the structure of 365-days of Fasting and Natural Living; a systematic way to master your health.

Become a Champion of Your Life. Take the Heal Thyself 12-week (4 semester) Purification and rejuvenation regimen that covers a span of 365-Days of complete Absolute Transformation and Wellness.

Natural Keys to Enhance Your Food Transformation

The key to success on this path of Purification is to experience 365 days of uninterpreted Cleansing as you take one day and one step at a time. Embrace foods of MAAT that bring balance, harmony, and wholeness, such as vegetables, herbs, whole grains, beans, nuts, seeds, sprouts and live juices.

Saturate yourself with chlorophyll, Green foods and juices, to overcome all ills.

Avoid foods of Set that cause disharmony and illness such as fried foods, flesh (beef, pork, chicken, fish), fast foods, Dairy, sugar, canned and frozen foods. Observe a 12-week Purification Program, 4 cycles of:

I.   21 Days of Natural Living
II.   21 Days of Live Food Cleansing
III. 21 Days of Juice Fasting
IV.   21 Days of Advanced Natural Living

IV is a combination of I-III cycles of cleansing and rejuvenation.

42 DAYS OF PURIFICATION
21-Days of Live Food Cleansing

Massage Treatment
Daily Exercise & Meditation Sessions
Soul Sweat
Colonic and enemas
Follow enclosed suggestions
Level II - Live Food Cleansing
60 %-70 % Wellness

21 DAYS OF PURIFICATION
21-Days of Vegetarian Natural Living

Heal Thyself Shut-In for each seasonal change
Daily Exercise & Meditation Sessions
Natural Food Preparation
(Follow recipes enclosed)
Soul Sweat
Colonic and enemas
Follow enclosed suggestions
Level I - Natural Living
40 %-60 % Wellness

Divine Maintenance To Establish A Natural Life Style
The inner sphere of the wellness universe represents 12 weeks (1 season) of uninterrupted cleansing for 75% to 100% cleansing and rejuvenation. The outer sphere of the wellness universe represents 365 days; a full year of cleansing and rejuvenation to experience 100% wellness. You must complete 4 seasonal Wheels to complete your 365 days, which will transform you into pure light.

63 DAYS OF PURIFICATION

21-Days of Live Juice Fasting

Massage Treatment

Daily Exercise & Meditation Sessions

Soul Sweat

Colonic and enemas

Follow enclosed suggestions

Level III - Juice Fasting
70 %-80 % Wellness

84 DAYS OF PURIFICATION

21-Days of Advanced Natural Living

Daily Exercise & Meditation Sessions

Natural Food Preparation (Follow recipes enclosed)

Soul Sweat

Colonic and enemas

Follow enclosed suggestions

Level IV - Advanced Natural Living
80 %-100 % Wellness

"Pass It On" for Nation and Global Building through Purification.

Every season, make a goal to "Pass It On" with someone in your life.

The more people you bring through on this mission of purification, by your example, the greater your power and transformation.

Supporting others through their transformation will encourage and strengthen you as you move on your wellness journey. By sharing wellness, it will assure you massive success, power and grace in your life. What goes around comes back around. Give that you may receive: First to yourself then to others.

A FASTER'S LETTER

From One Who Was Inspired to Share Her Wellness

This letter was sent to Loretta Threatt's six sisters. Loretta graduated from the Heal Thyself 21-Day Fasting Program that was given in Staten Island at the Sandy Ground Historical Society. Loretta's natural healing experience was so successful that she wanted to share with her family the blessing of self-transformation.

GREETINGS!

To: My Blood Sisters
From: Your Sister Loretta

Dearest Sisters: Several months ago, I attended Queen Afua's Heal Thyself 21-Day Fast for Cleansing and Rejuvenation of Body, Mind and Spirit, summer workshop. For those of you who are not familiar with her, Queen is the Director of the Heal Thyself Purification Center, located in Brooklyn, NY.

She travels the country teaching and sharing her many years of experience in the healing of the Body, Mind and Soul. She, herself, is the product of natural healing, and has, over the years, developed a 21-Day Fasting Program.

I participated in the 21-day Fasting Program and, as a result, evidence of my attendance was quite visible, as many of you noticed. Thank you for your compliments. You wanted to know what I was doing, and wanted me to share my experience with you, and that's exactly what Queen wanted and instructed her students to do! ! ! PASS THE WORD, LIBERATION through PURIFICATION!

Queen Afua believes that once our body Temples are purified we become liberated Body, Soul, and Mind. Once we receive our wellness blessings in order for us to maintain our results in a mighty way we must share the teachings of Heal Thyself with our love ones.

So, now sisters, if you are serious, and ready for your transformation, allow me to schedule the first wellness meeting for you. At this meeting, we will go forward with a 4 consecutive week schedule. Now, if you are ready note the meeting date on your calendar and I'll see you then. Bring A Donation.

Eternal Blessings,
Your Sister,
Loretta

FORMING A FASTING GROUP

Heal Thyself Do-It-Yourself Fasting Workshop Guide is for those who are not Heal Thyself Fasting Instructor Ambassadors, but have a desire to help others in need of wellness to form a support group for fasting within their family, spiritual house or community.

If you are one of these who are so inspired to pass on your wellness experience, such as Loretta Threatt did with her family, you can follow and organize a 1-day Community Fasting Shut-In or the Weekly Fasting Workshop with the guidance that is presented in the following pages. You and the other students of fasting can apply the information contained within this book. The following information will give you the format on how to execute a 1-day Fast and 21-Day and 12-Week cleansing group fast. Fasting and Natural Living Certification Training is available for those who desire to do this work professionally through the Heal Thyself Center.

The Beginning
One-Day Community Fasting Shut-In

The Heal Thyself One-Day Community Fasting Shut-In and the 21-Day Fasting and Live Food Cleansing Program is a most powerful transformative opening to a renewed life. In this new millennium, the mighty wake-up call of Liberation through Purification rings strong across the nation for it's a peoples' movement towards mass healing. As an answer and response to World Healing and Peace, we, of Heal Thyself, welcome you to the Path of Purification. The doors open for the masses to emerge onto the One-Day Community Fasting Shut-In as a first step to wellness. The Shut-In is a symbol for resurrection of absolute healing in body, mind and spirit, which unifies and gathers people from all walks of life.

As of March 22, 1996, Heal Thyself Housed in Smai Tawi; Afrakan Cultural Wellness & Meditation Center sounded the drums as the doors opened to the first Shut-In of this kind. One hundred and ten (110) people, all dressed in white, came forth to claim and celebrate the Afrakan Natural Life style Zone for world peace and healing through fasting and purification.

I have been leading the Fasting Crusade to reach out to every home, organization, spiritual center, corporation and educational institution; to every people, to every nation, encouraging fasting use as a necessary step toward personal and collective world healing. The Natural Living methods of Heal Thyself will not only heal the people who inhabit the earth, but will heal Nature itself. The time is approaching us. It is very near. This is a mighty, wake-up call; can't you hear? It does not matter what your religion is or what your philosophy is; it is purification that will set you free.

The ancients from every spiritual path left us a Divine legacy to fast and pray, that we might break every yoke, to unlock our inner prisons to set us free from dis-ease: socially, emotionally, physically and soulfully.

Violence, racism, greed, wars, natural disasters, mental break-downs and modern-day plagues are running rampant upon the earth due to consistent fall-outs of unnatural toxic living. We are bombarded with fast foods, violent media exposure, man-made poisons in our environment, the use of drugs, alcohol abuse and cigarette consumption, all resulting in societies' ills. We are truly in need, more than at any time before, of fasting and prayer.

Stop it all! No more toxic living, in words and deeds; for a One-Day fast will allow you to learn a new revitalizing, but ancient way, of living that will lay down the foundation for a whole new beginning. Don't give up on yourself. Give yourself another chance, a greater opportunity. Don't settle for an unfulfilled life. Rewrite your script into a live, Dynamic, Natural Way.

The doors to the One-Day Fast open at 9:30 a.m. During this time, sisters and brothers are registering for the days activity of self-healing. Others are receiving their first tonic for the morning, which is the Kidney/Liver Flush, made of garlic, lemons, cayenne, distilled water, olive oil and castor oil; just like Grandmother used to make. The fast begins at 10:00 a.m. and ends at sunset.

During the several hours that we are gathered together, Fasting Volunteers aid and support the attendees by answering the many questions as they hand out Wellness Literature and serve the various tonics that evolved from this inspirational day. Throughout the day, attendees will be educated on Natural Living and Fasting Techniques from Queen Afua and Baba Heru (Sen-Ur Semahj), an ancient Afrakan Nubian Priest. Baba Heru will bless the day with ancient Afrakan prayer and healing words of inspiration. Local Holistic Practitioners, within the Natural Healing Community, will render teachings on meditations, healing movements, colon cleansing, massage therapy, fasting methods and knowledge on foods and herbs that heal will be shared.

Throughout the One-Day Fasting Shut-In, we collectively pray, meditate, and affirm wellness as we lift our voices in Healing songs to further re-dedicate and establish in our lives a natural life style. As the day is done, and certificates are rendered, and hugs are exchanged, we all agree to Pass the Healing on. Those who are ready for intensive wellness will embark on the next step, the 21-Day Fast. Others will proceed to The Natural Wellness Program. All will leave, uplifted in the spirit of Liberation through Purification, to move onward at one's spirit-driven pace.

To all those who are touched by the One-Day Community Fasting Shut-In: May your light shine that it may spread throughout the world as you unfold into a more natural, loving, balanced, healthy, and spiritual being. In keeping with our Ancient Afrakan Spirit, under the banner of Heal Thyself, we bathe ourselves throughout this great day in Maat (representing balance, harmony, truth, justice, righteousness and wholism), as we collectively proclaim: I have the power to create in my life what I want it to be. Purification is the key!

"Pass It On"
Queen Afua

Basic 1-Day Community Fasting Shut-In
(For the Non-Certified Fasting Facilitator/Guide)

If you are unable to attend the Heal Thyself One-Day Community Fasting Shut-In at our locations in Brooklyn or Washington D.C., but you do want to experience a fasting Shut-In in your local area; you need the following seven elements in place.

Element 1: Gather speakers in Holistic Health who can share their experiences in Wellness, as lecturer or demonstration presenter on a volunteer basis.

Element 2: Prepare 4 Tonics/every 2 hours, on the hour:

Tonics for Purification	*Tonics for Rejuvenation*
• Kidney/Liver Flush	• Master Herbal Formula
• Fresh Fruit Juice	• Chlorophyll Drink

Element 3: Set Time of Shut-In. Either as early as sunrise, 6 a.m. to sunset, beginning with meditation and prayer, or begin when the Heal Thyself Center begins at 10 a.m. ending at sunset, 5 p.m.

Element 4: For continued wellness growth, use the One-Day Fasting preparation, as a jump-off into the 21-Day Fast. To prepare for the One-Day Fast, each participant should avoid for 3-7 days flesh foods, starches and fried foods; consume either fresh fruits, vegetables and/or herb teas according to need and drink one quart of distilled water every day with the juices of 1-3 lemons or limes.

Element 5: Secure appropriate location. Try to get space free of charge, such as community center, your job, a spiritual center or your home.

Element 6: Participants: Invite family, friends, co-workers, or the larger community, etc.

Element 7: Donations: Ask each person to bring a particular tonic or the dry materials to prepare the tonic. Some may bring a gallon of distilled water while others bring cups. Have a juicer in place to prepare fresh juices after or before the gathering begins for all to partake.

Promotion:

- Mail out Shut-In flyers to welcome friends, family and the general public.
- Sound the drum by word of mouth, speak out to everyone you meet, ask them to come and join in at the Shut-In.
- Put a message on your answering machine, telling of the date, location, time and fee.
- Speak to private or public groups, or family and friends about the Shut-In.

The Day has come. The Shut-In doors open. Hand out Fasters Purpose Statements to each one who gathers to be filled out. This activity will help participants to draw their prayer request to themselves.

Fasters Purpose Statement
To be filled out at the beginning of
the 1-Day Fasting Shut-In

Name: _____

Date: _____

Purpose Statement: _____

_____

_____

_____

_____

_____

_____

_____

_____

_____

_____

_____

_____

Dates of Results: _____

Place Your Statement in a Sacred Place.

Wholistic Self-Inventory Chart

Before you begin your wellness journey, please fill out this form so that you may have a reference to draw from. For if you don't know where you came from, you won't know where you are going, nor can you truly appreciate your wellness progression over the next 84 Days into holistic living.

Toxic Food Check List

Indicate Your Daily Food Intake as You Strive towards 100% Wellness

Do you consume any of these Food-stuffs. (Check even if taken in moderation). Indicate how often you consume these foods or engage in these practices within a week or a month.

FOOD	21 Day	42 Day	63 Day	84 Day
Meats: Pork, Beef, Chicken				
Chicken				
Fish				
Other Meats:				
Starches				
Dairy				
(Milk, Cheese, Ice Cream, Eggs)				
Sugar				
Coffee				
Fried Foods				
Fast Foods				
Late Night Eating				
Eating & Drinking Together				

Date: ___/___/___   Date: 365 Days ___/___/___

EYES, EARS, NOSE & THROAT	21 Day	42 Day	63 Day	84 Day
Asthma				
Colds				
Earache				
Enlarged Thyroid				
Eye Pain				
Hay Fever				
Hoarseness				
Gum Trouble				
Nose Bleeds				
Nasal Obstruction				
Sinus Infection				
Sore Throat				
Tonsillitis				

Over Time and Devotion to your cleansing, you will release these toxic foods to the point where the symptom has cleared up. As you change from the eating of food from this toxic list, then you will, in kind, begin to clear the dis-ease that you've checked off in your wholistic Self-Inventory Chart.

GENITOURINARY

	21 Day	42 Day	63 Day	84 Day
Bedwetting				
Dryness				
Frequent Urination				
Kidney Infection				
Painful Urination				
Prostrate Trouble				
Hysterectomy				
Alcoholism				
Drug Addiction				
Anemia				
Previous Surgery				
Cancer				
Cold Sores				
Diabetes				
Eczema				
Emphysema				
Epilepsy				

SKIN

	21 Day	42 Day	63 Day	84 Day
Boils				
Bruise Easily				
Dryness				
Itching				
Skin Eruptions (rash)				
Varicose Veins				
Fever				
Polio				
Stroke				
Ulcers				
Venereal Diseases				
Whopping Cough				
Heart Disease				
Measles				

FOR WOMEN ONLY

	21 Day	42 Day	63 Day	84 Day
Tumors				
Cyst				
Vaginal Itch				
Cramps or Backaches				
Hot Flashes				
Irregular Cycle/Infertile				
Miscarriages				
How many?				
Lumps in Breast				
Menopausal symptoms				
Painful Menstruation				
Vaginal Discharge				
How Many Days				
a month for Menses				

MUSCLE AND JOINT

	21 Day	42 Day	63 Day	84 Day
Arthritis				
Bursitis				
Foot trouble				
Hernia				
Low Back Pain				
Neck Pain & Stiffness				
Poor Posture				
Spinal Curvature				

Are you taking medication?

If so, what kind?

For how long?

How often?

For what purpose?

Indicate any other Health problems:

List on separate sheet

Sample Flyer for Shut-In

Heal Thyself One-Day Seasonal Fasting Shut-In
for Renewal of Body-Mind and Spirit

Date: _____

Location: _____

TONIC PRE-BREAKFAST Kidney/Liver Flush Tonic

10:00 - 10:30 AM	Morning guided Meditation/Heal Thyself Prayer
10:30 - 10:45 AM	Fasters state their purpose/Song: "To the Utmost Heal Thyself"
10:45 - 11:00 AM	Welcomes Mission Statement
11:00 - 11:30 AM	Colon Cleansing For Wellness

TONIC BREAKFAST- "REGENERATIVE HERBAL TONIC SONG" Heal Thyself Purification Prayer

11:30 - 12:00 PM	Fasting for the Spring - Fasting Presentation 21-Day Fasting Orientation & Live Food Cleansing
12:00 - 12:30 PM	Basic Massage and Reflexology for Stress Management
12:30 - 12:50 PM	Intermission for registration for Heal Thyself 21-Day Fasting Program
12:50 - 1:00 PM	Village Announcements

1:00 - 1:45 PM   Establish Natural Living for Total Wellness: Review Heal Thyself text

TONIC - GINGER JUMP TONIC - 2:00 Song: "I Have the Power"

2:15 - 3:00 PM   Viewing of Holistic Video and Discussion

Song: "Give Thanks and Praise"

3:00 - 4:30 PM   Community Holistic Healing Practitioner. i.e. masseur, masseuse, colon therapist, nutritionalist will offer presentation on holistic health.

DINNER TONIC - Green Power And Aloe Drink

4:30 - 5:00 PM   Graduation Ceremony/Includes Village Testimonial /Community Re-dedications/Purification Oaths

Closing

For the Healing Village · Visit Heal Thyself Shop for Products · Visit all Vendors · Enjoy Vegetarian Food for a reasonable fee · Meet with Your Heal Thyself Fasting Instructor for Personal Preparation and Registration for the 21-Day Cleansing Fast

Please wear White.

Heal Thyself 1-Day Fasting Shut-In™

Giving Up My Secret Formulas (Group)

Formulas are to be Presented Every 2 hours on the hour of the Shut-In.

- Use distilled water when Participants call for water;
- Prepare ingredients fresh, whenever possible;
- Use 1 gallon of solution per 30 participants.

Serve 10:30 A.M. Formula 1 — *Kidney/Liver Flush* an immune system builder

- 1 gallon of warm water
- Add 7 freshly squeezed juiced (organic) lemons or limes to break up mucus congestion.
- Add 1 cup of cold-pressed olive oil or Heal Thyself Inner Ease Colon Formula 3 to flush out the colon.
- Add to solution, 2 ounce bottle of liquid Kyolic (garlic extract) or 1 whole garlic, clove peeled, to eliminate bacteria in the system. Blend or juice garlic, then pour into water, lemon/lime and oil.
- Optional: Add ½ teaspoon of cayenne pepper for circulation.

Serve 12:00 Noon. Formula 2 — *Master Herbal Formula for Detoxification*

- 1 gallon water.
- Use Heal Thyself Master Herbal Formula (13 various cleansing and rejuvenating herbs).
- Boil a gallon of water the night before, then turn water off and add 4 ounces of herb tonic to hot pot.
- Allow to steep overnight.
- Strain and place in container the next day. Leave at room temperature. (Do not reheat or refrigerate)

Fasting volunteers should begin serving water by 12:00 noon or when a faster calls for additional water. Fasting volunteers are to be mindful to serve distilled water throughout the event, particularly to those who feel any discomfort i.e. headaches, dizziness, fatigue or itching or if experiencing mood swings. The Heal Thyself Breath of Spring formula also is offered throughout the event for more effective breathing. Offer this formula at the beginning and the end of the Shut-In.

Serve 2:00 P.M. Formula 3 - *Ginger Jump -Up Tonic*

Provide 1 gallon organic apple juice freshly pressed for circulation and energy.

- Add 1 cup of freshly pressed ginger root. Stir and drink.

Serve 4:00 P.M. Formula 4

- 1 gallon of distilled water.
- 1 pint Aloe Vera for cleansing.
- 1 pint liquid chlorophyll 100 mg. (green power) for rejuvenation.

The Breaking of the 1-Day Fasting Shut-In

Okra Recipe

- Ceremonially Pass okra for each one to receive.
- Bowl of raw okra.
- Add cold-pressed olive oil, salt-free celery salt, and powdered sage
- Dr. Bronner's seasoning to taste.
- Wheatgrass should be available for sale, in 1 ounce containers to be taken with distilled water at afternoon break, or at end of program.
- Suggested cost for the event could be anywhere from $10 to $30 per person, which then covers location materials, formulas and promotion of events.

Items should be purchased by Thursday and prepared by Friday, to be ready to serve by Saturday morning, to be ready and in place for the Shut-In.

Vegetarian Sample Menu

Breaking the 1-Day Fasting Shut-In.™

Tabouli Dish with Okra and Sage as a seasoning

Coleslaw (Graded purple and green cabbage with carrots and beets)

Garden Green Salad with Sprouts and Soaked Sunflower Seeds

Vegetable Juice and Wheatgrass

Live Food Dessert (i.e. sliced watermelon and cantaloupe and honeydew melon when in season.

For more recipes, see Chapters 7, 10 and 11 in this book and Chapters 4 and 7 in *Sacred Woman Guide to Healing the Feminine Body, Mind and Spirit*.

Now that we've done the Shut-In,™ it's time to move on through the Heal Thyself (4) levels of natural living and purification for a pain-free, invigorating, holistic way of living

Beginners Level I   21-Day Natural Living   21 Days

Level I is a transitional, natural way of eating that aligns one to a balanced holistic life style. Level I assists one in bridging a toxic-filled diet to natural food alternatives, that are nutritionally sound and supply the body with all the vitamins, minerals, proteins and calcium needed to build strong, cleansed body Temples. Natural living includes 50 %-75% live, uncooked raw foods and 25%-50% steamed foods.

Intermediate Level II 21-Day Live Food Cleanse   22-42 Days

Level II is a highly electrically charged natural way of eating, which includes 100% live food intake. The age-old concept here is that "Life begets Life," so as a result every bite you consume rebuilds and purifies you. Also Nature through the sun's rays, naturally and holistically, prepares our food from the fires of life. By eating live fruits and vegetables, grains, nuts, seeds, juices and herbs, we feed our tissue cells nature's pure oxygen, which gives us completely radiant health.

Advance Level III   21-Day Juice Fast   43-63 Days

Level III Juice Fast helps one take complete charge of his or her life by ingesting 100% liquids in the form of vegetable juices for rejuvenation and fruit juices for detoxification as well as herbal tonics with large amounts of distilled or spring water. Our body Temples are made up of approximately 75% water; therefore, by ingesting large amounts of water in these natural forms (i.e. juices), we are able to make tremendous strides in our body, mind and spirit transformation.

Heal Thyself Way of Life Master Level   64-84 Days

You have acquired good health now; but can you keep it? Say Yes! to 100% wellness. This level is the inclusion and incorporation of levels 1, 2, and 3 for the sole purpose of stabilizing and maintaining excellent natural health.

The details of this cleansing level appears in Chapter 9 and 10.

The Common Threads

Note that: For best results, all (4) levels include internal hygiene i.e. enemas and colonics, Heal Thyself nutritional and herbal formulas for cleansing and rejuvenation, healing salt baths, sweat baths, clay application and other natural cures, as well, for wholistic support.

Heal Thyself Valedictorian

365 Days of Natural Living! One year of following the Heal Thyself method of wellness will offer you a totally renewed body Temple on every level and will secure your future. You will experience renewed tissue cells, blood and bones, needed weight loss, renewed relationships, greater prosperity, balanced careers, harmonious love in your life, radiant skin and a more divine inner spirit.

Purification Success Team

Establish a Purification Success Team as you travel through 12-Weeks and 365 Days of Natural Living.

The Purification Success Support Team is a team that is created by each individual devotee of Natural Living. The team may include the following:

- Colon Therapist
- Masseur/Masseuse/Reflexologist
- Body Conditioner, Dance, Egyptian Yoga or Ari Ankh Ka, Egyptian Yoga Instructor
- Meditation Guide
- Numerologist
- Spiritual Counselor
- Health food or juice bar preparer
- Astrologist
- Natural Food Teacher

If a group of fasters will be using the above services, then you could create a package. If everyone in the group agrees to use the services 1-4 times during the 21-Day Fast or 12-Week cleanse or even throughout the year, than each practitioner might render a 10-20% discount for each service or product from said group.

Fast Level III

Fast and Cleanse from the following:

- All solid food;
- Violent, aggressive people and/or people who are not supportive of you healing yourself;
- Negative, violent Television and loud, aggressive Music;
- Adverse conversation, i.e. gossip; and
- Whatever is blocking your blessing, release it as you purify.

Heal Thyself 12 Week Purification Program

Observe 12 Weeks (84 days) of Purification To Perfect Wellness.

42 Days of Purification	63 Days of Purification
Level II - Live Food Cleansing	Level III - Juice Fasting
60 - 70 % Wellness	70 - 80 % Wellness
Date: _____/_____/_____	Date: _____/_____/_____
Weight Check in: _____	Weight Check in: _____
Record Your Successes During This Period:_____	Record Your Successes During This Period:_____
_____	_____
_____	_____
_____	_____
_____	_____
_____	_____
_____	_____

21 Days of Purification	84 Days of Purification
Level I - Natural Living	Level IV - Advanced Natural Living
40 - 60 % Wellness	80 - 100 % Wellness
Date: _____/_____/_____	Date: _____/_____/_____
Weight Check in: _____	Weight Check in: _____
Record Your Successes During This Period:_____	Record Your Successes During This Period:_____
_____	_____
_____	_____
_____	_____
_____	_____
_____	_____
_____	_____

I _____ vow to commit to living the Natural Principles of the Path of Purification.

Beginning Date: _____/_____/_____.

Signature _____

Supporting Witness

_____

Date _____/_____/_____

Home Healing

Are You Doing Your Homework? Your home should be a place of rest and comfort, a place of rejuvenation and peace. Your home should be your sanctuary, your temple or healing center. To make this a reality, one must avoid violent television-viewing, arguing in the home, physical abuse of husband against wife or verbal abuse of wife against husband or parents against children or children's disrespect to elders. The kitchen in the home must become a kitchen healing lab; the natural pharmacy of the home that produces a healthy family, and the bathroom must become the hydrotherapy room where water surgery and therapy is performed in order to avoid premature aging, early death, hostility, and diseased bodies. Each day that we cleanse ourselves of our negative ways and purify within our homes, we and our families radiate brilliant wellness.

Weekly or Bi-Weekly Support Meeting Workshops

Establish Bi-Weekly fasting support meetings that can go from 1½ to 2 hours. Always schedule workshops on the same day, same time, once the schedule is established.

Suggested locations: Community Centers, Spiritual Centers, or share space in each participant's home to save in cost of space.

An Example of a Support Meeting/Workshops

1. Recite Heal Thyself Purification Prayer.
2. Open purification discourse and sharing of healing testimonials. Each person expresses their goals for cleansing and discusses what challenges/victories they experienced weekly. *(3 – 5 minutes.)*
3. Sharing of Holistic Health Insights: Offered from 1-2 participants at each meeting on information from health magazines, outside workshops, and books outside of list. *(15 minutes.)*
4. Pick a chapter from *Heal Thyself* weekly to discuss. *(10 minutes.)*
5. Wholistic Recommended Readings, to be read and discussed *(30 minutes)* from the following list.

Book Reviews Listing:

Meeting 1-4: *Heal Thyself for Health and Longevity* by Queen Afua

Meeting 5-6: *African Holistic Health* by Dr. Llaila O. Afrika

Meeting 7: *Colon Health: Key to Vibrant Life* by Dr. Norman W. Walker

Meeting 8: *Mucusless Diet Healing System* by Arnold Ehret

Meeting 9: *Vitamins and Minerals from A to Z* by Dr. Jewel Pookrum

Meeting 10: *The Yoga of Nutrition* by Omraam Mikhael Aivanhov

Meeting 11: *Sugar Blues* by William Duffy or Dick Gregory's *Cookin' with Mother Nature*

Meeting 12: *Survival Into the 21st Century* by Viktaras Kulvinskas

6. Kitchen Power Circle

- Each student should bring a Vegetarian Pot Luck Dish or Healing Tonic.
- See recipes (Chapters 10 and 11) enclosed as a guide to Pot Luck Dishes or Tonics. Protein recipe with TVP/soy meatless product. Dairy-Free.
- Sugar-free and dairy-free desserts are welcome!
- Create a Meditation and/or a Prayer to overcome your food addiction as a collective (5 - 10 minutes.)
- Purification Affirmations. i.e. Heal Thyself Declaration of Independence.

Shout Out

"Liberation Thru Purification" to the four directions.

Ongoing project; Every 21 Days share with group your mandela and healing vision.

If you would like further guidance on facilitating a fasting or Natural Living Program, and further Natural Food Vegetarian visual guidance, you can order your Wholistic support Videos from Heal Thyself Center.

There are seven teachers who guide you on food preparation within the "Kitchen Power Video" and who assist in expanding your knowledge on the fact that food is medicine. It is advised that you study weekly from the video course, to strengthen your knowledge in the Kitchen Healing Lab.

The Birth of The Soul Sweat™

I've been sweating for many moons; seeking to find that still quiet space of inner peace while living in the city.

For over 20 years, I have frequented Native American Sweat Lodges as a form of natural healing and spiritual empowerment, which inspired me to bring forth the 'Soul Sweat.' Throughout the years, I took my children, friends, and clients with me to experience this powerful form of healing by indigenous people of Turtle Island.[1] I have been on the path of purification and natural healing since my teenage years and since that time I have healed myself of several diseases within my body. After years of sweating at the New York City bathhouse, my eczema was arrested and my skin has been glowing ever since.

I wanted to share my healing with others so that they could sweat out the poisons that we name as dis-ease. After discussing this with my husband, we decided to share what I named as the 'Soul Sweat,' a system of cleansing and sweating that was centered around various hot rooms that would detoxify the entire system on a physical, mental, and spiritual level.

It is the attitude, which makes a 'Soul Sweat™' work. As you enter the Soul Sweat (steam room) to detox, one visualize one's life-cleansing through the element of fire. See yourself burning up negative thoughts, actions, attitudes, and conditions. You're purifying your life on a soulful level. Surrender, your deep-seated hurt, anger, and rage with each prayer, herbal tonic, live juice, healing song and breath you take as you sweat your soul, body and mind into alignment. As you drink lemon water, and sweat, your inner pool is purified, yes, soothing the fire within, leaving you with a sense of calm and serenity. As you sweat, you drink green juice and herb teas to rejuvenate and repair tissues, cells, nerves, and bones. As you perform this work of healing, know that you are reconstructing and rebuilding your body Temple to its original form of Divinity.

Allow your addictions to purge out through your skin, the largest organ for elimination in the body.

---

1 The original name for America (in English) before it was renamed by Europeans.

My husband and I began visiting the Bath House several years ago to heal ourselves and share quality time together. After about one year of sweating and detoxing together, I began to create an organized system of sweating to detox the body, mind and spirit.

Together, we took many groups through the Fire and Water Transformation. The following layout is what was presented to thousands and, now, I am offering this system to you to detox yourself, your circles of family, friends and community.

Step Into the Mighty Soul Sweat

The *Soul Sweat* can be done with as few as two or as many as the space you choose to Sweat will allow.

Recite in Unison:

Opening affirmation and Heal Thyself declaration of independence:

"I have the power to create in my life what I want it to be; purification is the key...."

Tonic For Circulation:

Step 1   Blend together.
                ¼ cup of ginger juice
                1 pinch of cayenne
                1 lemon (juice)
                1-2 cloves of garlic
                16 ounces distilled water/serves 1-2

Step 2   Use 2-3 drops of Breath of Spring to purify your lungs and sinus

Step 3   Perform Fire Breathing 100 rounds (equal to) 3-5 minutes.

Step 4   Stretch the body through exercises presented in Chapter 17 for 15-20 minutes to release stress.

Step 5   Shower to activate and open up pores for quick sweating.

Step 6   Take a Sauna/Castor oil bath 10-15 minutes. (Freely apply pure castor oil over your body, from your scalp to your feet to draw out poisons. While in sauna, to keep charged and fully inspired, recite: "To the utmost Heal Thyself, I can Heal myself and turn my life around. I am Healing as I heal myself." Visit our Soul Sweat to learn the songs firsthand. Ralph Carter, my dear friend and profound artiste, wrote our first Heal Thyself song and sang it on many occasions in the bath house in New York as we ushered thousands through the Soul Sweats.

Step 7   While sweating each one present is to verbally Affirm what they are to release from their life, which is negative, and Affirm what she/he will bring into their life, which is positive.

Step 8   Shower from head to toe; drink master herbal tonic and green vegetable juice with one ounce of wheatgrass to empower and stabilize yourself.

Step 9   Take a Steam bath for 10-15 minutes. As you sweat, put legs up against the wall in a 45 degree angle, then massage arms, legs, hips, abdomen and chest. While self-healing, your Soul sweat leader presents a call and response of The Heal Thyself Healing Water Prayer. (That appears below.)

Step 10   Shower with hot and cold water; then drink a ginger and apple juice tonic for energy.

Step 11   Apply clay pack from head to toe, but, particularly, over the liver. Rest or meditate for 15 minutes or until the clay dries to draw out the toxins through the skin. (Shower.)

Step 12   Now, go back into the steam or sauna for 10-15 minutes; close out with a soap scrub for your final shower. (Use black soap or clay soap.)

Closing Prayer
Soul Sweat Leader

Recite the Ancient Afrakan Nile Valley Purification prayer of protection that apply in these times:

May I be protected by 70 purifications. I purify myself at the great stream of the galaxy. That which is wrong in me is pardoned and the spots on my body and upon the earth are washed away. I come that I may purify this soul of mine in the most high degree.

Seven

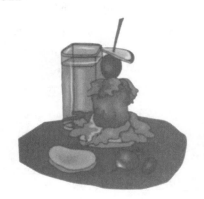

Life After Nutritional Fasting

Fasting gives you new opportunities and opens you up to new and greater possibilities. Fasting forgives, releases, enhances, restores, builds, flushes, washes, cleanses, and purifies us and all our relationships. Embrace yourself fully today; experience new beginnings, a new inner world, a healthier, more power-filled life.

WHEN YOU ARE coming off a 7- or 21-Day Fast, the return to solid foods must be gradual. Some of your old, eating habits will change, according to how often you fast and cleanse. Be prepared to give up heavy foods as you progress with each cleansing.

It takes 2-4 weeks to come off the fast properly. Avoid eating too much, too heavy or too late in the evening to prevent sickness or constipation in the morning. If you break fast too quickly, you may experience nausea, dizziness, depression or anger. You may even regain lost weight, experience bloating, tiredness or aches and pains. Avoid over-processed, hard to digest foods such as meats, fried foods, sugar, dairy and "junk food."

Incorporate these additional points in your normal health and maintenance program after any fast.

- Take vegetable juice 1–2 times daily.
- Take nutrients two to three times daily, i.e. spirulina, wheatgrass, green life.
- Take 2 enemas each week. While fasting take enemas daily or no less than 3 times a week and/or take an herbal laxative each day of your fast.
- Allow yourself 15-30 minutes of exercise daily.
- Take salt baths 1-3 times a week with 1-4 pounds Epsom salt or Dead Sea salt; omit if you have high blood pressure. Instead take a warm bath and soak 20-30 minutes.

If aches and pains persist, or swollen areas, you can continue to apply clay to affected area or the area that needs nurturing. Refer to section on clay pack.

Breaking A 7-Day Fast

Day 1 Eat only vegetables, raw or steamed.

Day 2 Include fruits in diet.

Day 3 to 6

Include vegetarian proteins. For meat eaters, include baked, unshelled fish and whole grains, but eat only in very small portions.

(One protein for the day, which could include sprouts, tofu, beans, peas and lentils, and one starch for the day, which could include tabouli, couscous, millet, brown rice, toasted whole grain bread etc.)

Day 7 **For the advance seekers of wellness,** discontinue starches and all proteins except sprouts.

Breaking A 21-Day Fast

Week 1: Days 1-2: Eat vegetables; steam them for 3-4 minutes. Also eat a vegetable salad. Consume as much okra as possible for it has a natural laxative effect.

Days 3-7: Include fruits. Eat a grapefruit each day. Do not eat bananas until two weeks after the fast is over. When you do,

make sure the bananas are well-spotted, as they will be in a
state that is easier to digest.

Week 2: Include small portions of vegetarian protein, such as lentils,
peas, beans (Soak overnight and prepare with ginger or bay leaf
for better digestion.), sprouts, eggless soymeats or miso soup.
Eat plenty of vegetables, raw and steamed, with proteins.

Week 3: Include whole-grain starches, such as couscous, millet, bulgar
wheat, tabouli, brown rice, and sprouted whole grain toasted
bread.

Week 4: If you have a great desire to eat flesh, eat baked fish. No
shellfish, chicken, beef, pork or lamb. Avoid all dairy products
from cows or goats such as milk, cheese and ice cream. Use
almond, sesame or soya milk and tofutti as a calcium source
instead. Also, eat green leafy vegetables and drink oatstraw,
dandelion and alfalfa herb teas.

You should take a week to break the fast, then either go into
live food eating or natural living, which includes minimal,
lightly steamed vegetarian dishes.

After fasting, it is advisable, in order to maintain your level of
wellness, to avoid starch or eat it once a day midday in small
amounts.

I've found that it takes at least a season to heal, but everyday that you
devote to healing yourself will get you closer and closer to your
wellness goal. Generally, we begin to study at the onset of a season, for
instance, from September to December or January to April. Through
many years of observation, I've found that it takes a season of
uninterrupted, self-healing to truly "Heal Thyself."

If after you have successfully completed your wellness season and
you decide to return to low-vibration, poisonous foods, your body will
react by detoxing immediately in the form of a runny nose, coughing,
headaches, dizziness, pain, rage or depression. You have outgrown
lower levels of food consumption. The toxic reaction indicates that you
have risen to higher levels of your health. You have a great deal of light
and vitality stored up within your body Temple. Therefore, you repel
disease-forming matter and can no longer participate in lower ways of
living.

So, if you have reactions from New Year's egg nog, 4th-of-July's fried chicken or the family reunion's sweet potato pies and collard greens stewed in lard, "run for your life" to the hydrotherapy room (bathroom) in your home. Hurry! Take an enema and healing bath so that you may return swiftly to your natural state of total health. As you purge from deep within your being, "bless your diseases away."

How To Deal With Minor Setbacks

Regardless of what happens, stay in a loving space. Be your best friend. Encourage yourself to grow beyond all odds. Healing your life is an ongoing process of self-discovery, self-observation, self-reflection, so be patient as you purify. Some days you will be right on point. Then, a life trial enters in: you're under pressure at work, or you encounter a family challenge. Everything that could happen, has, and you begin to react; old, unhealthy habits die hard. You reach for comfort. You grab for something familiar. So, you reach for mother's milk in the form of ice cream, if lonely and unfulfilled; or you reach out for the comfort of cookies and cake. You're overwhelmed and angry so you reach out for crunchy snacks and I'm not talking about celery and carrot sticks; you go for the hard-core stuff—"junk food." In your 'low-state,' you reach for a 'quick fix,' or a toxic way of handling your emotional state and reactions from the trials of life. You believe toxic food is the answer, but I assure you, it's not and never will be. If you find yourself caught up in negativity, before you know it, then study yourself in the midst of your toxic consumption and observe how you feel, why you feel that way, and what you can do to resolve your inner emotional conflict even as you eat toxic food. Your answers are between you and what you are about to consume. On this path of purification, strive to release guilt and learn from your lessons—for guilt engenders destructive behavior. We are in a process of reconstruction. Regardless of what state of toxicity you find yourself in, you can overcome, over time.

It takes time to build up cravings in your body for toxic food. Most time the desire is passed down in your food from one generation to the next. You were, in most cases, born with a predisposition to certain foods due to your parent's food consumption. You're made up from the joint toxic foods and the cravings and thoughts that your parents embodied. In order to break the cycle of toxic foods that, ultimately, leads up to a continuation of family dis-ease, i.e. a family who suffers from high blood pressure, diabetes, respiratory problems, cancer, fibroid tumors in women, or prostrate conditions in men, we must detox wholistically over time with conscious, loving effort, steadily adapted to a natural life.

Setbacks:

- If you fall off for one meal, don't miss a beat. Jump right back into a large salad or a green juice, as your next meal to balance you out. Study what situation challenged your emotions and begin to rectify your emotions and feelings with prayer, affirmations, deep breathing and journaling.
- You may have eating buddies who work against your having healthy eating habits. It's time to circle yourself with people who are striving to be positive, progressive, healthy people who will draw out the best in you.
- Develop patience for your ups and downs and, overtime, you will have more ups and fewer downs as you journey through a season of detoxification and rejuvenation.
- Take one meal and one day at a time; you will win in the end.
- Give thanks for each successful day of natural eating or juice fasting.
- Celebrate your wellness success every 7 or 21 days. Take yourself out to the theatre, or visit your favorite museum or go to a poetry gathering, or sit down to a candle-lit vegetarian meal with yourself and/or a love one.

Preparation is the key!

Consider the very real probability of the family reunion, wedding, or holiday dinner and, then, consider the fact that if you do not prepare for yourself and the other people with special dietary needs by encouraging the family to have a few vegetable or whole grain dishes included in the menu, you will find yourself challenged in maintaining your natural living practices. You may be delving into foods that send your blood pressure skyrocketing i.e. meats, greasy foods etc. that send you into a state of anxiety or depression from sugar-filled cakes.

- Love yourself, no matter how deep you fall.
- Pull yourself up; let's try again! You'll do better next time.
- *Constipated:* If constipated, take a herbal laxative, as soon as you get home, consisting of senna and mint or cascara sagradra (3 tablets) or aloe ¼ teaspoon to a cup of water. Perform this 1—3 days straight or take an enema with lemon and water.
- *Emotional Stress:* Take a 1 pound hot Epsom salt or Dead Sea salt bath for 30 minutes as you release the emotional anxiety from foods ingested or unbalanced emotions due to your participation.
- *Hyperactivity:* To counteract hyperactivity or stress due to sugar consumption, take 50 mg. of B complex for 7 days and take ¼ teaspoon goldenseal with 8 ounces of water.
- *High Blood Pressure:* If you're eating heavy foods and your pressure goes up, take 1-2 cloves of garlic with the juice of a lemon and 16 ounces of warm water enema before going to bed.

Next time if you're going into a non-vegetarian food camp, then be sure to have a healthy vegetarian meal at home before going out so that you don't get caught up in the madness because you're hungry.

Non-Stop, Uninterrupted Natural Healing for Success

Within every two-week cycle, your body Temple will progressively build upon itself. By the time you reach the 1,000 Lotus Petals, Crown Chakra or Divine Wisdom Center located at the top of your pyramid, complete healing will be accomplished. Alternate for 12 weeks beginning with 7 days of Natural Living followed by 7 days of Nutritional Fasting. Study and follow the instructions given in this chapter as your guide.

Once you've reached 12 weeks of Purification, you have now moved into the portals of higher living.

In accomplishing this three-month, self-healing process, you will be liberated from addictive, poisonous foods, drinks and smoke. You will then be able to accept freely the *7/7 System* as a way of life.

Food is your medication — *"Eat to live; don't live to eat."*

Note: This program does not diagnose or prescribe. If under a doctor's supervision, please continue with medication until you are over the dis-ease.

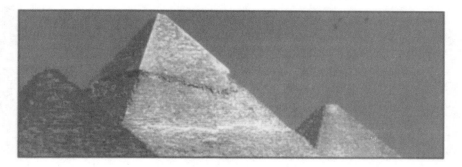

Human Pyramid Power

The pyramid in the first civilization represented the living body. They were built to house the afterlife of the king and queen who were the embodiment of the nation. The pyramid housed the best of our nation in human form. The pyramids were built as an earth portal from which our ancestors could ascend to the spiritual plane and, thus, travel to the Light of Divinity. The pyramid was built by the hands and spirit of a collective consciousness of priests and priestesses, engineers, and healers like that of Imhotep, by stone masons, plasterers, brick layers and officials.

> The pyramid temple from the 1ˢᵗ to 4ᵗʰ Dynasty was built as an offering to Ra (the light) to ensure the continuing cycle of rebirth of the underworld from the earthly realm to the underworld. — *Egypt The World of The Pharaoh* by Dorothea Arnold.

The king and queen rested and were reborn within the upper room of the pyramid that represented the nations' ascensions. Divinity was conferred on the king and queen in the upper chamber of the pyramid, enabling the nations' ascension and ensuring the past, present, and future evolution of the people. Our Ancestors experienced a spiritual rebirth within the highly charged pyramids when their bodies died. I believe we can experience and perform similar natural miracles and rebirth ourselves within our living bodies; all this through the internal healing journey of Healing Thyself while on the natural living program of Heal Thyself. This wellness journey aids us in moving from a dead state of dis-ease to be reborn into an alive state of wellness through consistent devotion, love, and divine discipline for our resurrection.

The pyramids were technically constructed in perfect symmetry to elevate the health of the people physically and spiritually. The pyramids have survived longer than any structure known to man.

Today, we must emulate the past by restructuring our body Temples to a state of excellence. This is done through constant detoxification and the rejuvenating benefits to be gained from a year of consistent, uninterrupted seasonal juice fasting, natural living and the eating of live foods, which, in turn, promote internal hygiene. Surround yourself with supportive friends and family, who will aid you in overcoming your health challenges. Surround yourself also with skilled people to assist in the resurrection of your body Temple, i.e. masseuse, colon hygienist, wholistic health practitioner and others.

Every Step Goes Higher and Higher!
Three Months to Create a New You!

1. The pyramid represents: Enlightenment, Resurrection, Divinity, Wisdom and Illumination. As you step higher up the pyramid ladder, you become one of "the Shining Ones"—

    Peaceful, Pure, Powerful and Potent.

2. Use the *7/7 Three-Month Pyramid Program* on the onset of the seasons: spring, summer, fall and winter.

3. When the body is in an open stance, it takes on the form of the pyramid. The pyramid is a form that is used as a healing symbol of humankind striving toward perfection.

4. As you raise and energize your healing awareness, the Crown Chakra (energy center) awakens and, then, you are fully purified (healed) and spiritually realized (enlightened).

5. It can take 84 steps (days) to reach Cosmic Consciousness, which is 75%-100% self-healing, according to the Heal Thyself Method illustrated in this chart.

6. Six cycles (which is 12 weeks) gives you enough time to maximize and actualize your physical, spiritual, as well as business and romantic goals.

1ˢᵗ Approach to the Human Pyramid of Power

Three Month 7/7 Chart for Resurrection of Body, Mind and Spirit

Heru — the Divine Spirit within You

100% Healing = Enlightenment

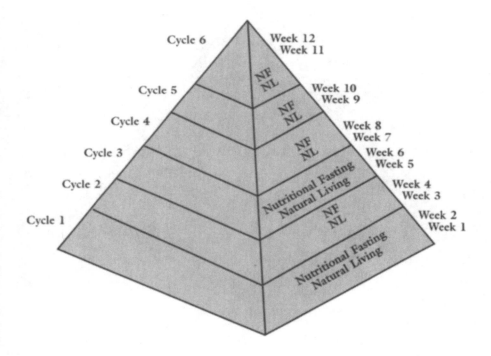

7 Days Nutritional Fasting   7 Days Natural Living

Code: Natural Living = NL (pure foods)
Nutritional Fasting = NF (juice fast)
Every 7 days, you alternate between NL and NF.

2nd *Approach to the Human Pyramid of Power*

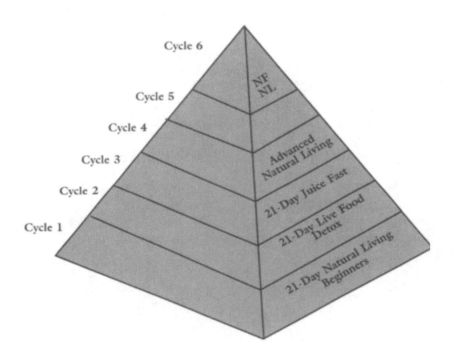

Every 21 Days Raises You Up higher as your dietary intake becomes more refined and your health becomes more and more illuminated.

This 84-Day Process of Wellness can take place over 4 seasons — a period of one year—to maximize results, and to gain life, healing and the ability to break addiction.

Nutrition and Alternative Foods

As is indicated throughout this book, the food we eat can either become our poison or our medicine. This list indicates the foods that you should avoid and which ones are preferable for health. Meat, dairy, processed foods and sugar cause most of the health problems that people experience. Removing them from your diet will improve your health, energy level, mood, and mental clarity. It may take a while to make all of the necessary adjustments, but you will see a noticeable improvement. For each of the foods on the low-vibration list that you eliminate, you will find yourself closer to a disease-free, healthy, vibrant and powerful body.

Foods To Avoid

The following list is of foods to be aware of and to avoid as you clean out your kitchen healing Laboratory and clean up your body Temple.

Meats: The purpose of meat in the diet is to provide protein. But, meat can cause infections, constipation, headaches, cancer and premature aging. We can, at best, consume vegetarian protein, that are not dis-ease provoking, such as beans, peas (kidney beans, black beans, soya beans), tofu, TVP, lima beans, lentils, nuts, seeds, sprouts and spirulina (sea algae). As a homework assignment, read *101 Reasons Why I'm A Vegetarian,* a paper put out by Vegetarians Society in New York City.

For personal empowerment, form a vegetarian support society with your community i.e. within your school, college and spiritual circle. Vegetarian support groups should share recipes, health videos and books. You can invite guests who can expound on the virtues of the vegetarian life style. Our children need strengthening against the challenges of well-meaning family and school friends who may pressure our children to go off their path of purification. When my children were younger, I created an organization called Clean Teens, for my eldest children that contained 16-20 young people and parents and the Young Sprouts for my youngest child that contained 7-10 children. Both children and parents were empowered to maintain a wellness life style, against all odds.

Sugar: Beware of sugar in the form of corn syrup, corn sugar, brown sugar or white sugar. Artificial sweeteners can cause hyperactivity, stress, bone deterioration, poor memory, loss of hair, and bladder cancer. The best source of natural sweets are fruits and the licorice herb that is called the sweet root. Alternatively soak dried fruit such as dates and raisins and use the water to sweeten your tea or your cereal, or to make lemonade rather than using sugar.

Salt: Salt (sodium chloride) is an inorganic mineral that can't be used by the cells in the body. It irritates the bloodstream and the stomach and blocks the digestion of food. Salt intake can cause high blood pressure, kidney and liver dis-ease. The best sources of salt (sodium) are found in celery, spinach, kale, carrots, lettuce and strawberries.

Fried Foods: Cooked, greasy foods clog up arteries. If your arteries stay clogged, overtime, you may experience cold feet and hands, sluggishness, heart palpitations, headaches, swollen ankles and hands and high blood pressure. If you have a history of addiction to fried foods, then drink lemon or lime juice with warm water twice a day. Also drink 8-12 ounces of fresh organic orange, grapefruit or pineapple juice every day with 12 ounces of water.

Starches: Eat only whole grains and whole foods, i.e. tabouli, bulgar wheat, couscous, baked potato, sprouted whole grain toasted bread, raw or lightly steamed corn on the cob in moderation. Avoid starches that are devitalized i.e. white rice, white bread, and white macaroni are difficult to digest. They clog up the colon causing constipation, which leads to 90% of our dis-eases, according to the late Dr. Robert Wood, a last great Colon Hygiene Practitioner and one of my teachers. A rule to observe with devitalized or whole grain starches; eat no more that a few spoons or ½ cup and accompany your starch with lightly steamed or raw green salad to help 'broom' out excess starch from your colon. Don't eat starch when the sun goes down, it will not be digested and, as a result, you will wake up the next day, fatigued, anxious and depressed.

Dairy: Dairy's role is to provide us with calcium for the growth and strength of our bones and is also supposed to calm and balance out our nervous system. But, dairy can cause allergies, asthma, hay fever, vaginal discharges, fibroids and boils to name a few illnesses that are derived from dairy.

Healthy vegetarian calcium can do the same healing, but without the negative side effects. So, it is best to consume almond milk, sesame milk, sunflower seed milk, soya milk, or 8-16 ounces of green vegetable juices 1-2 times a day. The vegetables that are high in calcium are broccoli, kale, spinach, turnip and wheatgrass. The herbs, that are high in calcium and are my favorites are dandelion, alfalfa herb and seaweed vegetable such as spirulina; use powder for best absorption. The recommended daily allowance for calcium is 800-1200 mg.

To Be Powerful

To be powerful is to be mighty, to be fully alive, to be in alignment with your divine self, to be centered, to be strong and potent in your day-to-day living. To be powerful is to have control of your thoughts, and your actions. In order to break toxic habits, you must grow into your power by overcoming the pull of the commoner, eating destructive, man-made food rather than naturally, Divinely made food. The clearer you are inside, the more naturally effective and mighty you will be in your life.

Our most Ancient Afrakan Ancestors from Smai Tawi, known as Egypt, said this in relationship to power and purity. "I am pure at a place of passage." "I have destroyed my defects." "I have made an end of my wickedness." "I have annihilated the faults which belong to me." "I myself am pure." "I am mighty." — *The Book of Coming Forth By Day* interpreted by Wallis Budge.

To be powerful, you must be the captain of your ship and direct your course by not succumbing to negative forces. To be powerful, you must be the King and Queen over your body Temple and maintain a healthy Temple through mastering and overcoming a dis-eased state of being, by aligning yourself with a natural way of living. To be truly powerful and reclaim your power, you must follow the laws of Nature to assist you in purifying self; thereby, becoming one with the Most High's Almighty Power.

Low-Vibration Foods: When you find yourself craving or consuming low-vibration food, usually, you are thinking of and behaving in a toxic state. Become conscious and purify consistently to break the addiction to toxic foods. When you take in low-vibration food, you also attract negative, obsessive, greedy, hostile, suppressive people.

High-Vibration Food: The quality of our foods dictates the quality of our lives. When you desire and consume high-vibration foods, your inner environment is vibrating on a high plane. Your foods, your thoughts, and actions reflect your high state of being, goodness and wellness follow you all the days of your life, according to the high maintenance of your vibration. When you consume high-vibration foods, overtime you begin to attract positive, loving, supportive, gentle, giving reflections.

Low-Vibration Food *(Foods to eliminate)*	*High-Vibration Food Alternatives* *(Recommended transitional foods)*
Cow's milk	Soy-, nut-, goat-, human-milk; kefir
Ice cream	Soy ice cream, tofutti
Cheese	Rennet-less, unsalted cheese or grated tofu
Margarine	Soya margarine
Yogurt	Brown Cow yogurt*
Eggs	Organic eggs*

* *Although these two items are listed as alternatives, try to eventually eliminate these foods as well.*

White bread	Whole wheat and cracked wheat bread (toasted bread)
Vinegar	Organic apple cider vinegar
Salt	Sea salt, kelp, dulse
Chocolate	Carob
Gelatin	Agar-agar (use to make 'Jello' with your favorite fruit juice)
Water	Distilled or spring water
Bottle/can juice	Fresh squeezed/pressed fruit juice
Peanut butter	Fresh unsweetened peanut butter
Junk food	Freshly prepared popcorn, brown rice cakes, dried fruits (banana chips, pineapple, apricots, raisins), banana custard, frozen juice (instead

Low-Vibration Food (Foods to eliminate)	High-Vibration Food (Recommended vital foods)
	of ices), chilled fruit, baked apples, blue corn chips, seaweed chips, whole wheat pretzels, unsalted potato chips prepared in sesame or olive oil.
Shellfish*	Fish with fins and scales (clean and garnish with fresh lemon to eliminate some of the bacteria). Eventually try to eliminate flesh foods altogether

*** Note:** *Shellfish includes lobster, shrimp, clams, etc. which are scavengers of the ocean. They eat waste in the ocean. When we eat them, we further poison ourselves.*

Deep/stir-fried	Steam food. Remove from flame. Add 1-2 tablespoons cold-pressed (uncooked) oil to food
White macaroni	Whole wheat macaroni
White rice	Brown rice
White flour	Whole wheat or barley flour
Other grains*	Millet, couscous, bulgar
*Corn flakes or 'sugar pops'	
Pancakes	Buckwheat, whole wheat, bran, flaxseed
Grits	Soy grits, barley grits
Oil	Cold-pressed olive oil
Cornmeal cereal	Whole oats, granola
Corn starch	Arrowroot powder
White sugar	Raw honey, maple syrup, blackstrap molasses, fructose
Protein:	
meat, poultry, fish	Sprouts, tofu, miso, seeds (sesame, pumpkin, sunflower), nuts (pecan, walnut, pistachio, almonds), beans (black, pinto, kidney, etc.), peas (black-eye, etc.) Also use soya meats as an alternative.
Canned/frozen vegetables	Fresh vegetables (steamed or raw)

Low-Vibration Food   High-Vibration Food
(Foods to eliminate)   (Recommended vital foods)
    Soda   Fresh juice, mineral water or distilled water

In the place of dairy (milk, cheese, ice cream), eat soya products. For calcium, almond milk, sesame milk or soy milk.

Note: *Eat whole grain starches only three times a week preferably during the hours of 12-4 p.m.*

Natural Vitamin Supplements

Calcium	Oatstraw and comfrey herbs, sprouts, carrots, green leafy vegetables, nut milk, and soya milk
Vitamin A & D	Carrots
Vitamin B	Yeast and bee pollen
Vitamin C	Rosehips herb tea
Vitamin E	Alfalfa, wheatgrass
Minerals	Kelp, other sea plants such as spirulina and blue-green manna.

Nature has provided us with a great variety of fruits and vegetables, beans and whole grains so that we need never be bored of eating simply and naturally. Remember to use organic, unsprayed fruits and vegetables whenever possible.

For further information, study *Nutrition Almanac, Prescription for Nutritional Healing*, by James F. Balch M.D. and Phyllis A. Balch, C.N.C.

Recommended Fruits

Sweet fruits	Pomegranates, bananas, dates, raisins, dried apples and dried apricots
Sub-acid fruits	Mangoes, peaches, plums, pears, green grapes, dark grapes, papaya
Acid fruits	Strawberries, raspberries, blueberries, pineapple, grapefruits, oranges, lemons, tomatoes, boysenberries
Melons	Cantaloupes, watermelon, honeydew melon (to be eaten alone)

Recommended Vegetables

Asparagus	Onions	Dandelions
Beets	Okra	Irish potatoes
Celery	Parsley	Lettuce
Cabbage	Greens of all kinds	Swiss chard
Cauliflower	Watercress	Spinach
Carrots	Parsnip	Beans
Cucumbers	Pumpkin	Squash
Turnips	Rutabagas	
Tomatoes	Sweet potatoes	

Starches   Millet, tabouli, couscous, corn-on-the-cob, bulgar wheat, squash, coconut, potato, yam

Seaweed   Dulse, nori, hijiki

Proteins   String-, green-, wax-, lima-, navy-, kidney-, soy-beans; split peas, lentils, chick peas, pigeon peas

Sprouts   Alfalfa, mung, and all sprouts

Nuts and Seeds   Almonds, walnuts, filberts, brazil, pecans, sunflower, sesame and pumpkin seeds

For those who want more information on food alternatives, go to *Heal Thyself Natural Living Cookbook* by Dianne Ciccone.

Avoid Mucus-Forming Foods

Mucus-forming foods contribute to many poor health conditions, such as colds, shortness of breath, fevers, hay fever, asthma, loss of hearing and sight, constipation, female disorders, (such as tumors, cysts, vaginal discharge, PMS) male prostate gland blockage, fatigue, weight problems and mental congestion.

To eliminate excess and unhealthy mucus from your body Temple, in the mornings drink freshly prepared juice of 2 grapefruits, 2 oranges and 2 lemons or freshly prepared pineapple juice. Due to concentrated levels of sugar in fruit juice, dilute equal parts of water to juice to avoid skin eruptions or mood swings.

In the mornings, you will expel mucus from nose, eyes, ears, vagina (if a woman) and anus. The more mucus that comes out of the body, the closer you are to returning to a disease-free body.

To support your cleansing further, take 2 herbal laxatives weekly until the problem is eliminated. Other methods include: senna and peppermint (1 teaspoon of each herb steeped for 1 hour), powdered aloe (4 teaspoons in water), cascara sagrada (1 teaspoon in water or 3 capsules), or *Heal Thyself Colon Deblocker* (3 tablespoons with lemon water taken 3 times a week).

Special Meals for the Person in Transition from Meat-Eating

Meatless Meals for Lunch and Dinner

1.) Soya meat (in place of turkey or fish), steamed broccoli with chopped scallions and a garden salad.

2.) Baked sweet potatoes, bulgar wheat "meatloaf" (bind with sugarless tomato sauce, onion, peppers and whole wheat flour) and a garden salad.

3.) Caribbean meal: Brown rice and peas (This is a poor food combination, but you may have it occasionally.) and steamed okra and onions to aid digestion.

4.) For picnics, serve barbecue tofu (Use a barbecue sauce from a health food store; it should contain no sugar or additives.) corn on the cob (Use soy margarine and dulse.) and Queen Afua's Rainbow Salad. (Find recipe in Chapter 10.)

5.) Southern meal: Black-eye peas, string beans, whole grain cornmeal corn bread (use any recipe, but substitute organic dates or raisins (soaked) or raw honey for sugar, egg replacer instead of eggs, almond, sesame or soy milk instead of cow's milk). *Note:* Include soaked flaxseed or a few tablespoons of bran to act as a laxative.

Eight

Hints for Natural Living and Fasting

Act Now!

MOST ILLNESSES ARE the result of shattered dreams, unfulfilled goals, and empty promises in one or many areas of your life. To change your karma (action and reaction), do things that make you blissful. Don't wait to live; this is all the life you have. Freedom and bliss await you at this very moment. Live every moment fully, as if it were your first and last.

As you develop this blissful state, the internal war that's going on within your body Temple that takes the form of disease begins to diminish, and your eating habits begin to reflect this process. What we eat relates to our state of mind. For example, when you eat and/or desire fried foods, you are usually angry or bitter. When you desire dairy, you are in need of nurturing. When you desire meat, you are feeling aggressive or you are attracting aggression to you. When you are consuming a great deal of starch, it is because you are feeling unfulfilled.

On a positive note, when you eat a lot of fruit, it brings out a sweet disposition and bright, beautiful thoughts. When you eat green vegetables, it brings out and reflects inner peace.

85

A Meeting With The Creator

Here's how I tap into the power zone of unlimited possibilities. Most of *Heal Thyself for Health and Longevity* revealed itself to me, during the hours of spiritual power and anointing; between 4:00 a.m. and 6:00 a.m. I rose from my sleep to enter the union of my left brain (physical and mental sphere) and my right brain sphere, the (spiritual and intuitive) union of balance and the center of Divine knowledge. Within this realm, a fluid flows from the pineal gland located between the eye brow and slightly above the eyes. The ancients called this spiritual center the uchat. This fluid renders you to a super state of higher awareness where you vividly hear the voice of the Creator speak through you. You are able to ask any question and the answers divinely usher from you, for you are in perfect union with the Creator where all truth flows. If one needs spiritual guidance in matters of career, love, healing, finances, relationships, or knowledge on how to overcome challenges, then for 7-9 or more nights avoid eating any solid foods once the sun goes down. To further sharpen your intuition and be in total union with the Most High, saturate your bloodstream with dark, green, vegetable juices throughout the day.

When I have life-altering questions, I rise at 4:00 a.m. and pray and meditate and remain still, I can hear the voice from within speak to me, then I drink 8-16 ounces of warm water with lemon or I drink herbal tea such as gota kola for the mind or dandelion for complete rejuvenation. I begin to breathe deeply into my heart center 50-100 times; until I completely relax and let go of any fear of truth revealing itself to me. I have found that most of the time when we are afraid of truth, what we are really afraid of is change; letting go of our unproductive painful patterns. If I am still blocked, then I'll go so far as taking a 2-4 pound salt bath. As my body drinks in the heated salt water, answers reveal themselves to me spontaneously. Oh happy day(s), I've gotten out of the way and allowed truth to rescue me as I meet with the Creator on this divine, early morning day.

The Ancients were Tapped In

The Nile Valley queen/king, priest and priestess wore the double crown of the consciousness Smai Tawi (unity) of left and right brain.

One side of the crown was white representing spiritual ascension and the opposite side was red, which represented power over the material realm. This level of inner unity represents an ascended master, one who is in total alignment with the Divine who is fully enlightened.

Today, as in ancient times, our mental, spiritual, social, emotional and physical survival is only attained by Natural Living Principles; much of what you will find within the passages of *Heal Thyself.*

Activities that help you to successfully develop self and support you on your path to purification and your cleansing life style:

- Join a health food co-op.
- Form a buddy system or support group.
- Become a member of a health spa.
- Visit a Turkish bath house.
- Take food preparation classes.
- Write or recite poetry.
- Take a mini-vacation once a month.
- Do poetry.
- Meditate.
- Go to the theater.
- Start your own business.
- Dance! Sing! Play! Act!
- Develop a natural healing and spiritual library.
- Have clay facials and clay baths with family members and/or friends.
- Take a field trip with your cleansing buddies to holistic and spiritual bookstores, crystal shops, health food stores and holistic health fairs.

Incorporate these activities into your life style and live by the Heal Thyself Purification Method to accomplish your goals and create success in your life.

Every season, you go through 84 days of wellness.

The system is as follows:

The One-Day Fasting Shut-In seasonal healing releases the old and takes on the new.

Perform:

- 21 Days of Natural Living
- 21 Days of Live Food Eating
- 21 Days of Juice Fasting
- 21 Days of Advanced Natural Living (a combination of the previous 3 levels as presented above, but with greater intensity) for the advance devotees of purification.

Follow the above wellness work over 84 Days; Repeat this for four seasons and your toxic, troubled condition will transform into the embodiment of the one Divine; thereby, the Netenu (Angelic Quality of the Divine) within you will become awakened, as you journey within the protective healing path of purification. You will once again walk the earth as giants amongst man and woman; and your good works and deeds will shine, throughout the world; as you carry within you the mantel of health and wholeness.

It will take 365 Days to establish a profound, transformative, natural life and to detoxify one's entire life. Four phases, four seasons of ongoing cycle of wellness is what is called for to gain body Temple restoration. The purpose of taking on 365 days of divine discipline and wellness and devoting yourself to purification is to detoxify one's entire life. This 365 day cycle will assist one in establishing a natural life style, that will aid in eliminating dis-ease and disharmony from the body and mind, leaving the spirit free. This intense resurrection/labor of love will cleanse your past karma (shai) of your previous evil-doing. As you travel and focus on purification through all the seasons, you will come to witness a complete change, as Khepera (transformation) aids you on the Path of Ra (light). Like the pyramids, "every round goes higher and higher."

Daily Affirmations for Higher Living

Depending on your religion, vocalize the name you use for Creator of the Universe.

1.) I practice forgiveness so that I, too, may be forgiven, for it is the will of the Creator.

2.) I practice thanksgiving in all my actions, thought and deeds, for it is the will of Allah.

3.) I will walk as gently as a deer and glide as smooth as a bird within the temple walls of my divine home, for it is the will of the Most High.

4.) My voice will be just above a whisper and only to be raised in states of divine joy and bliss, for it is the will of the Krishna.

5.) I will always strive to be patient, loving and giving for it is the will of God.

6.) I will serve graciously, joyfully, peacefully those in need, for it is the will of the Neter.

7.) As I begin fasting, I will give my food away to one, who is most needy, for it is the will of Yahweh.

8.) I will stay in constant prayer in all my thoughts, words and deeds, for it is the will of Olódùmarè.

9.) Whatever goodness I expect from others, I will first be that goodness myself, for it is the will of Jehovah.

10.) I will fast 24 hours weekly and 3, 7, or 21 days monthly so that I might be an example of the Creator's law, for it is the will of Jah.

11.) I will harm no living creature. I accept my vegetarianism. I will not use drugs or alcohol for I must keep my body so pure that I may be accepted in thy sight, for it is the will of Yahweh.

12.) I will purify all my words, thoughts, and actions for it is the will of Great-grandfather's and Great-grandmother's spirit.

21 Affirmations for 21 Days of Natural Living and Live Food Cleansing

Day 1   I am no longer angry at my disease. I am now able to "bless my disease away," for my disease has no power over me.

Day 2   I look forward to my healing. I look forward to my daily cleansing.

Day 3   I say *YES* to my personal success in gaining physical, mental, spiritual and economic harmony and abundant health.

Day 4   I liberate myself through purification.

Day 5   I accept 100% healing. I am disease-free; it is reflected in my life.

Day 6   I shape my destiny with each thought. I think thoughts of success, and know in my soul that nothing is blocking me from my good except myself. I have the power to remove all blocks with fasting and prayer.

Day 7   I release my excess weight in thought, word, body and deed.

Day 8   I live a full, happy life—without fear.

Day 9   Disease is no longer in my life. My cells, blood, bones, nerves, tissues and arteries are filled with pure joy.

Day 10   I am an inspiration for myself and others.

Day 11   I welcome each day with an open mind and an open heart.

Day 12   No one blocks me from my blessings but me. I release all my blockages and free myself.

Day 13   My purification is the key to my long, healthy and vibrant life.

Day 14   Today I am in perfect harmony with myself and the universe.

Day 15   May I continue to be a shining example of health and wealth in body, mind and spirit.

Day 16   Thank you, Creator, for allowing me to wake up to another day of living for I have another opportunity to make it right.

Day 17   I affirm that my reflections bring me love and joy this divine day.

Day 18   Today, I am whole and happy. The Creator is active within me and I am active within the Creator.

Day 19   Each atom within my being is being fed with life-giving juices, herbs and high-spiritual thoughts, so all is well within me. I give thanks.

Day 20   I am ecstatic about my healing.

Day 21   I accept purification in my life here and now and for all eternity.

Use the affirmations as spiritual treatments. Read the affirmations 3 times a day—at sunrise, midday, and sunset. As you breathe the affirmation in your soul and repeat it, the affirmation and you become one and the same.

Health Diary

Congratulations on the first day of the Heal Thyself Life Plan! Purchase a notebook or blank page diary. Fill in your day-to-day experiences. If at anytime during your cleansing you wanted to sing, dance, cry, write poetry, or shout for joy, then put it down in writing. Use these pages to express who you are, how you are, and what you desire to become. In other words, fill these pages with your very being.

Later, the pages will come to reflect your purification experience as a term of growth; a daily chapter in the book of yourself, showing your development from embryonic stages on through to your ever-blossoming rebirth. Review diary at the beginning or at the closing of your day. Whenever you're ready to begin your self-healing, that is a good time to begin your review.

You can use colored markers to express your experience for the day. You will see a rainbow chart of your cleansing life. Apply this color system during your fasting or natural living program.

BLUE	for a peaceful, balanced day. Harmony
RED	for increased energy and power. Challenge
PURPLE	for spiritual experience and inner harmony.
BLACK	for normal day, business day. Discipline.
PINK	for love experience of self or another.
GREEN	for healing experience, financial blessing received.

Life Goals to Affirm While Cleansing

While on your cleansing and purification path, look at all areas of your life in which you want to see a change. Fill in this form or note in your diary with all the goals you wish to achieve. Include as many of these areas as you can, along with whatever else you hope to gain from fasting. Ask And It Shall Be Given. So Be It. Continue on this cleansing plan—until your goals have been reached.

Family/Home Life Goal:

_____
_____
_____
_____

Relationship Goals:

_____
_____
_____
_____

Health Goals:

_____
_____
_____
_____

Personal/Development Goals:

_____
_____
_____
_____

Business/Professional Goals:

_____
_____
_____
_____

Financial Goals:

_____
_____
_____
_____

Keep record of all the things you have asked for and note the day
and time you received your blessings.

Weight Loss Goal

Record Your Progress

Cycle I—1ˢᵗ day	**Cycle III — 28ᵗʰ day**
Date: _____	Date: _____
Present Weight: _____	Present Weight: _____
Weight Goal: _____	Weight Goal: _____
7ᵗʰ day	35ᵗʰ day
Date: _____	Date: _____
Present Weight: _____	Present Weight: _____
Weight Goal: _____	Weight Goal: _____
Cycle II — 14ᵗʰ day	**Cycle IV — 42ⁿᵈ day**
Date: _____	Date: _____
Present Weight: _____	Present Weight: _____
Weight Goal: _____	Weight Goal: _____
21ˢᵗ day	49ᵗʰ day
Date: _____	Date: _____
Present Weight: _____	Present Weight: _____
Weight Goal: _____	Weight Goal: _____

Supporters

As you cleanse, you will notice that your supporters become more supportive and even your non-supporters become supporters. Then, you can place them on the supporters list or they will leave your life, for you have cleansed that lower part of their reflection out of your life. As you yourself become a loving supporter of yourself, then and only then will all of life support and love you. The wind, the rain, the sun and snow will all embrace you, for you are pure in heart, body and spirit. You will say, "Dear Creator, may we all be good reflections of you as we, humbly, follow your natural laws of living."

Below make a list of your supporters and non-supporters and why they either support or oppose what you are doing. Next to their name write the color they make you feel like when you think of them. See how that color in them changes as you move deeper into your cleansing.

SUPPORTERS

Name: _____

Why: _____

Color: _____

*Remarks:*_____

_____

Name: _____

Why: _____

Color: _____

*Remarks:*_____

_____

Name: _____

Why: _____

Color: _____

*Remarks:*_____

_____

NON-SUPPORTERS

Name: _____

Why: _____

Color: _____

*Remarks:*_____

_____

Name: _____

Why: _____

Color: _____

*Remarks:*_____

_____

Overseas Travel Health Kit

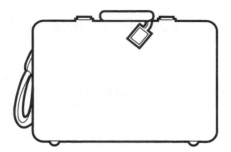

Don't leave home without it!

- When traveling, you sometimes find yourself not eliminating as usual. To prevent constipation, take a quart-sized enema bag or herbal laxatives for cleansing once or twice a week. Keeping your body light will add ease and enjoyment to your trip.
- To maintain a healthy, immune system, take powdered spirulina, which contains protein, calcium, vitamins and minerals. Use powder rather than tablets for easier digestion. Take 1-2 tablespoons two times a day to strengthen your immune system and protect against weakness and disease.
- To heal from internal bleeding or heavy menstrual flow, take Shepherd's Purse 1-2 tablespoons to 2 cups of water.
- Carry a few lemons until you are able to purchase some in the local market to avoid congestion from colds and respiratory imbalances. Simple lemon water helps one to digest foreign foods.
- A small, citrus juice extractor (saucer-sized, manually operated) in order to squeeze fresh orange, grapefruit, lemon and lime juices.
- Goldenseal powder for infection. Use 1 teaspoon in warm water two times a week to protect against infections as it keeps the blood pure.
- Carry spiritual reading materials, to help you maintain your mental and emotional center.
- Lecithin for circulation and memory.
- Vitamin B-Complex, to maintain a calm nervous system.

Tropical Traveling *"DOs"* and *"DON'Ts"*

Don't Eat:

- Fried Foods — they clog arteries, which leads to poor circulation, and poisoned blood which results also in red eyes.
- White sugar or cooked honey — they cause poor memory and nervous tension. Sugar eats up the nervous system as well as the bones, which results in tooth decay and arthritis. Use raw honey, whenever possible, instead of white sugar.

Do Eat:

- Breakfast

Breakfast Alternate

Juice of 1 lemon, cayenne and 1 cup of warm water.

Freshly squeezed orange juice, using 3-4 oranges.

Freshly squeezed grapefruit juice, using 2 grapefruits.

Fresh fruit, i.e. papaya or watermelon.

Oatmeal cereal, 3 times a week. Use raw honey; let it soak in hot water 3 minutes. Don't cook to avoid constipation.

Lunch and/or Dinner

Coconut water and its meat.

Twenty minutes later, eat any leaves (vegetables) and okra soup (use fish, okra, peppers, tomatoes, onions).

Boiled bananas, not fried (Watch out for constipation.).

If fish is used for protein, limit to 1-2 times a week and boil or steam, instead of frying. Seek out beans, peas, lentils or nuts—for vegetarian protein is your best choice.

If you must have starches, take them with lunch or before 7 p.m.

Yams, fufu 1-3 times a week (eat okra on your heavy starch days to keep your bowels open and clear).

Rice 1-2 times a week; soak rice before cooking or even better, overnight.

Bread may be taken every other day unless you have constipation, then avoid bread and starches.

Peanut soup or raw peanuts (ground nuts): soak minutes before eating.

Do Remember:

We should have at least 2-3 bowel movements a day for excellent health. If you have only one movement a day or few times a week, then eliminate all starches for 14 days. Remember, we carry 5-20 pounds of old, impacted waste that has accumulated in the colon over the years.

Salt Baths

Take full body or foot baths at least once a week.

Stay in tub for 20 minutes while massaging body from feet to head.

Ocean Baths

While in Afrika and the Caribbean, ocean and salt baths are a special gift and should be taken as frequently as possible.

Sand Baths

Dig a hole big enough to bury yourself in; cover yourself with the sand. Bathe inside the "Earth Mother" for 30-60 minutes while re-charging from the sun. Exit from sand and rinse in the ocean. Emerge from the Healing Water. Stretch out on the sand as the sun cooks life into your body Temple.

This bath is excellent for cleansing the poisons from the system, beautifying the skin and drawing you closer to your Maker.

Nine

Natural Living: with Juice Fasting

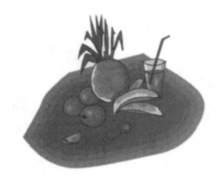

Recommendation for Divine Living

Rejuvenation + Purification = Harmony in Body, Mind and Spirit

Rejuvenation =   Vegetables (live and steamed), chlorophyll, wheatgrass and spirulina; rejuvenating herbs.

Purification =   Enemas, herbal laxatives and colonics; purification herbs; fruits.

Levels of Mastery

Freshman   Organically fed chicken and fish (not shellfish) baked or broiled; 75% steamed vegetables, 25% raw vegetables. *Whole grains*—brown rice, bulgar wheat.

Sophomore   Soya meats, beans, peas, nuts, seeds and sprouts. 50% steamed, 50% raw-vegetables. *Whole grains*—brown rice, bulgar wheat.

Junior   Sprouts (alfalfa, mung and others). 25% steamed, 75% raw-vegetables. Light grains such as tabouli and couscous.

Senior	Live, uncooked foods and sprouts, which are a form of vegetarian protein. 100% raw diet of fresh fruits, vegetables, juices; nuts and seeds (eaten in moderation).
Master	50% of diet — juices and herb teas. 50% of diet — fresh fruits and vegetables. No grains, nuts or seeds.
Ph.D.	A "Ph.D." purified diet would consist of 100% Live vegetarian consumption with pure air and pure water as your support. Alas, we have cleansed the planet, by starting from within.

Level I, II and III Natural Living Diet

(Alternate with the Nutritional Fasting Diet as a Natural Life Style)

Pre-breakfast:

(*This is to be taken two times a week only*).

Juice of one lemon with 8 ounces warm water.

Up to 2 tablespoons of cold-pressed olive oil with drops of Kyolic or 2 tablespoons of the Colon Deblocker.

The pre-breakfast is to be taken upon first rising, and at least 30 minutes before eating or drinking or anything else. Its purpose is to enhance the cleansing process that the body experiences during sleep. The lemon juice helps to remove mucus. The cold-pressed olive oil lubricates the colon and facilitates elimination. The garlic, or Kyolic (an odorless garlic extract) cleanses the blood and adding cayenne (not recommended in cases of high blood pressure) improves circulation.

Breakfast:

Vegetable or fruit juice

1 tablespoon Queen Afua's Super Nutritional Formula

1-2 pieces of fruit (Give yourself 30 minutes to 1 hour between eating and drinking)

Note: Each food group requires a different digestive juice. If you bring two different juices together, the digestion becomes impacted and shuts down or digests food incompletely. The result of poor digestion

is blottiness, gas, constipation, and a distended abdomen.
Don't combine the following:

- Eating and drinking don't combine
- Fruits and vegetables don't combine.
- Proteins and starches don't combine.

Combine the following:

- Vegetable and starches. i.e., greens and brown rice or tabouli, etc.
- Proteins and vegetables, beans, nuts, seeds or vegetables of any kind.
- Melon are to be eaten alone, i.e. cantaloupe, watermelon, honeydew melon, etc.
- Citrus is to be eaten alone, i.e. oranges, pineapples, grapefruits.
- Sub-acid fruits are to be eaten alone, i.e. apples, pears, plums, berries, etc.

Combination Juices:

- Ginger is flexible; ginger combines with fruits and vegetables.

Breakfast consists of 2 to 3 servings of fresh fruit, such as grapefruits, oranges, papaya, pear, 2 pounds of grapes, melons, particularly watermelons, plums, mangoes and cherries. If you eat bananas, they should be well-ripened with plenty of spots. Try to concentrate on fruits that have been specially recommended to you. Don't eat dried fruits because of the concentrated sugar that will destroy your teeth. After eating all fruit, brush with Queen Afua's Clay and a non-abrasive toothbrush.

Lunch:

Large raw salad with plenty of sprouts.
All sorts of green, leafy vegetables; do not steam for more than 3-4 minutes.

Vegetarian protein source; eat lentils, peas, sprouts, tofu or soya meats. T.V.P. (Texturized Vegetable Protein), soya chicken, soya turkey and soya beef.

Beans must be soaked overnight. However, do not eat more than

2 ounces of nuts or seeds. No peanuts or cashew nuts.

If you are not a vegetarian, you may eat baked or broiled fish, no more than 1 or 2 times weekly. No shellfish (lobster, clams, or shrimp).

Try to follow this only as a transitional diet until you become a vegetarian.

Add 1 tablespoon of Heal Thyself Super Nutritional Formula with juice.

Lunch should comprise a large salad, steamed leafy greens and a protein. The salad is made of raw vegetables. (Try to include plenty of okra.) Use a light salad dressing. No mayonnaise or other dairy products, please! Green leafy vegetables (kale, dandelion, mustard) can be steamed for 4-5 minutes.

You should eliminate all animal products (beef, chicken, fish, milk and other dairy products). You will get your proteins from lentils, peas, tofu, sprouts, and meat substitutes that are not made from eggs.

Natural couscous, millet, brown rice, and baked potatoes; eat them with vegetables for better digestion. Eat large amounts of green vegetables to assist in brooming out the excess starch that you've consumed.

One or more vegetable juice combinations have been recommended to cleanse and strengthen the body. This should be made with a vegetable juicer (not a blender) and consumed immediately after juicing for greater healing properties to be present.

Dinner:

Repeat lunch meal.

No protein or starch after 7 p.m. or after the sun goes down

1 tablespoon Super Nutritional Formula with juice.

Dinner is a repetition of lunch. All cooked food should be eaten before the sun goes down. Afterwards, eat live foods (raw fruits and vegetables). Drink one pint to one quart of distilled or purified water.

Avoid all fried foods and microwave cooking that destroys the live enzymes contained in life-giving foods.

Level III:

Nutritional Fasting (7-21 Days)

Fasting Preparation: For those who are going to pass Level I and II and go immediately into a fast, follow the following directions as not to suffer from extreme detoxing.

Greetings to fasters and champions of Purification who are ready to go the distance for New Beginnings, Peace and Empowerment, Cleansing and Rejuvenation. We welcome you to prepare for the 21-Day Fast.

Beware! If you have been poisoning your body Temple with toxic living for months or years, subconsciously or consciously, then prepare for at least the 21-Day Fast.

Please adhere to the following instructions on how to prepare for your Fast.

The more time you have to prepare for your fast, from as few as 7 to as much as 21 Days, the easier and more effective the fasting process will be, and the less toxic the reactions you will experience.

Preparation of at least three weeks is best.

Purification for Liberation

Degree I
Beginning students   75% vegetable juice, 25% fruit juice.
Degree II
Intermediate students   50% vegetable juice, 50% fruit juice.
Degree III
Advanced students   Fruit juices
                            Wheatgrass 4 ounces or more
                            Spirulina, 2-3 tablespoons three times
                            a day in 1 quart to 1 gallon of water.

It took me 16 years to master natural living and fasting as a way of life and diet. It is a process. Be sure to read how to begin and how to come off nutritional fasts in the *Fasting* section of this book. Above all, be consistent and patient.

Pre-Breakfast:

Kidney-Liver Flush: (blend together)
juice of 1 lemon
3 tablespoons Colon Deblocker
12 drops of liquid Kyolic, or 1-2 cloves of fresh garlic
1 pinch to ¼ teaspoon cayenne pepper
8 ounces distilled water

Breakfast

Fruit juice (8-12 ounces)

Lunch:

Vegetable juice (8-12 ounces)

(Vegetable juice must be prepared fresh for greatest potency. If you can't obtain fresh juice at lunch time, then drink fruit juice now and prepare the fresh vegetable juice for breakfast.)

1 tablespoon of Super Nutritional Formula with each juice meal.

A word to the wise: If you must prepare dinner for your loved ones while fasting, be sure to drink 12 ounces of vegetable juice with your nutrients before you begin preparing the meal to eliminate any desire to taste the food you are preparing. Drink at least 6-8 glasses of pure water daily.

During Levels 1 to 4, your daily or weekly routines should include: internal cleansing (nasal and colon), bathing, physical exercise and activity, drinking of Master Herb formulas, clay applications and spiritual meditations and prayer.

Internal cleansing: Enemas should be taken daily while on the Fast. Add the juice of one lemon to the water. (Also see the *Hydrotherapy* chapter). During period of Natural Living or Live Food detox, take 2 to 3 enemas weekly until well.

External cleansing: Baths—Use 4 drops Eucalyptus oil and 4 pounds of Epsom salts in a tub of warm water. (Note: Salt should not be used if you have high blood pressure. Use herbs and oils instead.)

Take baths 3 times a week. Soak body for 30 minutes and up to an hour if suffering from stress and high levels of toxicity. Massage body in an upward motion toward heart while in tub.

Enemas or baths should be taken 2-3 times a week over the next 12 weeks, or season of cleansing. Take a shower after bath. (Also see chapter on Hydrotherapy.)

Clay application   For major problems, use a clay pack with gauze overnight. For minor problems, use during day and evening hours. Shower off once clay is dry.

Physical activity   Review Chapter 17 of this book.

Tonics   Take the Master Herbal Formula 4-7 times a week to break addictions.

Preparation: Boil 4-5 cups of water; turn off flame; add 3 teaspoons of herbs to water and steep overnight. Drink in the morning.

Drink 1 pint to 1 quart of distilled water daily.

This is Your Time For Transformation.

Juice Recommendations

Drink up to a pint of Vegetable Juice every day for Deep Cleansing and Rejuvenation!

Vegetable Juice Combinations

Note: Take small amounts in the beginning to avoid a fasting "detox" reaction.

Carrot/beet   For blood cleansing and building: ¼, ½ or 1 whole beet and 1 or more carrots.

>   *Note: Don't use beets if you have high blood pressure.*

Cucumber, carrot, parsley For edema: to relieve water retention and aid in kidney healing. 1 or more carrots, ½ to 1 whole cucumber (remove skin, if waxed) and 2 bunches of parsley.

Carrot/celery   For relaxation (anti-stress): 2 stalks of celery and 1 or more carrots.

>   *Note: Don't use celery if you have high blood pressure due to high sodium content.*

Carrot/scallion To clear congestion from lungs. 1-2 radishes, 1 or more carrots and 1 teaspoon horseradish.

Carrot/ginger To increase circulation, 1 or more carrots with ¼ cup of freshly pressed ginger.

Carrot/leek   To eliminate high blood pressure. 3 or more carrots and 1-2 pieces of leek.

Carrot/turnip To relieve arthritis in joints: 3 or more carrots with 1 turnip. *This is a bone knitter.*

Carrot/cabbage For indigestion: 3 or more carrots with a quarter of a cabbage.

String beans and carrots For diabetes: 1 or more carrots and 2 pounds of string beans.

Pure green drink For body restoration, ½-1 whole bunch of parsley, a few sprigs of watercress, 2-3 leaves of kale and ½ of cucumber.

Note: Although carrot is high in calcium and vitamin A and D, it is still a hybrid vegetable. To aid in your transition to juicing, you may add 1-3 carrots to your other vegetables. Overtime omit the carrots and move into consuming Green juice for more profound rejuvenation.

Fruit Juice Combinations

Apple   Helps cleanse the blood. It acts as a natural laxative.

Pineapple   Fights congestion and helps remove mucus.

Cranberry   Helps fight cancer and cleanses the blood.

Papaya   Helps relieve indigestion.

Grapefruit/orange/lemon

                   Helps to eliminate respiratory difficulties, sinus congestion and vaginal discharges.

Grape   Helps cleanse the blood and aids the elimination of mucus-forming food residue.

According to the "Juice Man," you should wash fruits and vegetables with the juice of one lemon and a few teaspoons of sea salt (dissolved in a quart of pure water). Or use 2 tablespoons of Dr. Bronner's liquid soap diluted in 1-2 quarts of pure water. Be sure to rinse the fruits and vegetables with pure water.

For foods that have been waxed, such as apples and cucumbers, cut off the skin before juicing. Better yet, use organic fruits and vegetables grown without the use of poisonous sprays.

Introduction to Green Juices

Green Juices   Juices made from kale, spinach, broccoli, cucumber, watercress, etc. Juice anywhere between 8-12 ounces.

Green vegetable juices help to restore your blood, tissues, cells, nerves and bones. Green Juice is high in calcium and other minerals. Green juices balance out the emotional body. It reduces stress and anxiety as it gently purifies. Green juices prevent and eliminate dis-ease such as high blood pressure, mental depression, arthritis, etc. Green juice is a beauty tonic. It helps to create radiant, blemish-free skin, healthy hair, and clear eyes, free from redness and discoloration.

Ten

Recipes from Queen Afua's Kitchen Laboratory

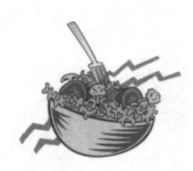

Food is our Medicine.

Rainbow Salad

½ shredded green cabbage
*½ shredded purple cabbage**
3 shredded carrots (for calcium and vitamins A & D)
1 shredded beet (cleanses and builds the blood)
Garnish with parsley around the salad

*Cabbage aids digestion; juice or eat raw.

Mix together with eggless mayonnaise from your neighborhood food cooperative or health food store and 3 tablespoons of soy sauce.

Do not use soy sauce if you have high blood pressure.

Berry Fruit Salad

2 cups of strawberries — sliced in half
1 cup of blueberries
1 cup raspberries
½ cup grated raw coconut
Garnish with 1 cup of chopped pecans.

This salad is excellent to cleanse the blood.

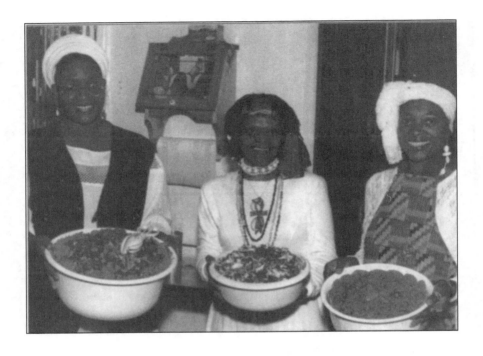

Garden Green Salad

1 head of lettuce*
1 bunch spinach (for iron)
1 whole red pepper (for vitamin C)
1-2 cups of alfalfa sprouts (a vegetable protein)
½ bunch of watercress
Sprinkle ½ cup of soaked sunflower seeds (optional)

*Do not use Bibb lettuce, for according to the late herbalist Dr. John Moore, it contains morphine.

Combine ingredients and serve with following dressing:

Cold-pressed olive oil (a colon lubricant) and apple cider vinegar (which breaks up mucus and congestion).

Sprout Salad

3 cups alfalfa sprouts
3 cups mung bean sprouts
½ cup chopped scallions
½-1 cup red peppers, sliced into strips

Combine the above with one of the following dressings:

Mix equal parts of olive or sesame oil and organic apple cider vinegar.
Add tamari sauce or Dr. Bronner's Soy Sauce to taste.

You also may use an oil and vinegar dressing (*without sugar or additives*) from your local food coop.

Summer Melon Salad

½ watermelon

2 whole cantaloupes

1 whole honeydew melon

Scoop out watermelon first to use as a "boat" for the fruit of all the melons.

Use a melon ball scoop to create a nice look for the salad.

This salad cleanses the water in your system and purifies the kidneys. Melons should not be mixed with any other foods.

Winter Fruit Salad

3 yellow pears (diced)
3 apples (diced, but remove skins, if waxed)
1 cup walnuts (soak for a few hours or overnight for greater digestion)
1 teaspoon cinnamon powder
4 tablespoons wheat germ (sprinkled over salad)

High Protein Nut Milk (Shake)

½ cup pumpkin seeds†

3-4 tablespoons tahini butter

1 ripe banana

Maple syrup or blackstrap molasses (for iron)

1 tablespoon lecithin (brain food)

† for restoration of male reproductive organs

Combine in blender. Drink and enjoy.

Note: You can also use almonds, brazil nuts, pecans, sunflower seed. Always soak nuts and seeds.

Ginger Drink (For Improved Circulation)

1 cup of juiced ginger (for digestion and circulation)

3 lemons or limes (for vitamin C and mucus elimination)

Maple syrup or raw honey

Blend 1 quart purified water with ingredients.

Heat slightly during winter months or drink at room temperature.

Tofu Egg Rolls without the Eggs

*2 cakes of tofu — mash to a cheesy consistency

½ cup miso or 3 tablespoons tamari/soy sauce with ¼ cup water

1 cup sprouts (mung bean or alfalfa)

2-4 grated carrots

Pour off any liquid after you've blended the ingredients.

Lay flat 3-4 sheets of Nori seaweed on wooden board.

Put in 2 cups of mixture on the sheet and roll together in the shape of an egg roll. Slice in half.

* Note: Beans are converted into tofu, which means they automatically go through a cooking process.

Tofu Pizza

Pizza Spread — *grated tofu (create a cheese-like texture), natural tomato sauce (without sugar) or blend 2 tomatoes and 2 teaspoons Italian seasonings*

Put a little soya margarine on sprouted whole grain bread and then use tofu pizza spread.

Eat a large side order of kale, spinach, okra, or broccoli with any and all starch meals.

Tofu on a Bed of Tabouli

Tabouli is a light and easy to digest grain that does not require cooking; thus, it produces very little mucus formation or congestion in the body. It's low in calories.

Soak 2 cups tabouli in ½-1 cup of warm water for 15-20 minutes

Add chopped scallions

1 whole onion

⅓ cup steamed okra†

2 tablespoons sage*

*Don't use sage if breast-feeding. It dries up the milk.

† For a laxative effect, which will "sweep out" the system in a few hours.

Add other herbal seasonings that you so desire.

Once prepared, place tabouli on a plate or platter.

Dice 1 cake of tofu, (Crumble the high protein soybean curd to give it a textured look.) with your desired seasonings in the center of the tabouli platter.

Garnish around the tabouli with parsley (high in iron) to be eaten with this dish.

Easy Cereal

Couscous and oats as a cereal — to be eaten only 1-2 times a week.

Soak 1 cup of grain in 1 cup of water for 15 minutes.

If you cook these grains rather than soak them, you will become constipated.

Add cinnamon, nutmeg or raw honey as a sweetener.

A half to 1 hour before eating any grain, drink warm water with lemon or fresh vegetable/fruit juice.

Non-Dairy Ice Cream Dessert

Freeze a couple of peeled bananas and 1 cup of strawberries.

Once the above ingredients are frozen, chop up and put in blender.

Add 2 teaspoons cinnamon or nutmeg, 2 cups walnuts, and sugarless vanilla (from the health food store).

Add ½-1 cup of almond or sesame milk depending on consistency desired.

For ice cream sandwiches, spread the combination over a rice cake. Sprinkle coconut over the spread and then place a second rice cake over the coconut.

Put in plastic bags and then in freezer to have ready whenever you would like a healthy dessert for you and your children.

Making your Heavy Meals Light

Whenever you prepare a bean or vegetable bean soup, add one of the following after the soup has been completely prepared:

1 cup of diced okra. Add to soup or salad

1 teaspoon of cascara sagrada, or *3 tablespoons with 12 to 16 ounces of water or 1 tablespoon flaxseed* (soaked overnight).

Blend flaxseed with apple or pear juice.

These in a soup once or twice a week will help to avoid constipation.

Bean Soups

Black beans, kidney beans,
pinto beans, black-eye peas,
aduki beans, lima beans.

Always add vegetables of your choice to your bean soups.

Steep the vegetable in the soup for 5-8 minutes. Then the soup is ready to enjoy.

Soak the beans overnight for less cooking time and less gas accumulation.

Cook beans for 45 minutes to 1 hour.

Cook in a cast iron or stainless steel pot.

To eliminate gas from beans, prepare beans with cup of ginger juice, or when beans are ready, put a handful of ginger bark, cut up, and add to soup while cooking or use 3-4 pieces of bay leaf.

All beans can also be sprouted for raw-food eating.

Check your public library or health food store for an easy-to-follow booklet on sprouting.

Marinated Vegetables with Tofu Chunks

1 cup of sliced or diced red onions
1 cup of sliced white onions
1 cup snow peas
1 cup broccoli
Diced tofu
2-3 tablespoons tamari sauce, or to taste
Sage or other herbs that you enjoy

Marinate the ingredients for a few hours or overnight.

Serve on a bed of green leaves and garnish with red or yellow peppers.

Avocado Dip

2 ripe avocados
2 cups of unsweetened tomato sauce
or 2 chopped tomatoes
2 tablespoons miso (fermented soybeans), or Dr. Bronner's soy sauce
2 cups water

Blend and place in a serving dish.

Place celery and carrot sticks around the tray to use as a dipper.

For heavier eaters, use blue corn chips or seaweed chips.

Five-Minute Laxative Soup

*3 cups okra**
1 cup parsley (high in iron)
½ cup leeks and/or onions (good for high blood pressure)
1-2 cups vegetable bouillon
1 teaspoon cascara sagrada (tablets)

Note: Cascara sagrada can be found in health food stores or co-ops.

* Acts as both laxative and rejuvenator for genitals.

Add the above ingredients with 3-4 cups of water.

This soup takes 5 minutes to prepare.

Uncooked Desserts

Uncooked Pie Crust

2½ cups ground sesame seeds
2 tablespoons sesame oil
1 teaspoon raw maple syrup
1 tablespoon warm water
1 teaspoon natural vanilla extract

Mix with hands and press into sesame-oiled pie pan.

Pie Filling 1

2 chopped pears (remove skin)
2 chopped apples (remove skin)
½-1 teaspoon cinnamon
2 tablespoons maple syrup
¼ cup raisins

Let the above ingredients marinate overnight.

Spoon onto pie crust and top it with 2 tablespoons of wheat germ.

Decorate with well-ripened sliced bananas and sliced strawberries.

Pie Filling 2

1½ cups sliced strawberries
1½ cups blueberries
1½ cups raspberries

Combine ¼ cup of each berry with ¼ cup water and 2 tablespoons maple syrup.

Blend and pour over the remaining berries that have been put in the pie crust.

Cover with ½ cup freshly grated coconut and ½ cup chopped walnuts.

Other resource food/cooking books include:

Cooking with Mother Nature by Dick Gregory

Heal Thyself Natural Living Cookbook by Dianne Ciccone

The Book of Whole Meals by Anne Marie Colbin; and

Complete Vegetarian Kitchen by Lorna Sass.

Eleven

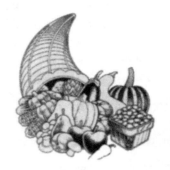

Afrikan-
Caribbean Meals

I am a firm believer that "You are what you eat," and "Your health is your wealth."

NAJAMI LEZAMA HAS been a massage therapist, fasting therapist, and exercise instructor, involved in the performing arts for over 20 years. She is now working in the healing arts and conducts massage workshops for adults, children and babies. Najami has taken my Heal Thyself students and devotees of wellness to teach them over the years how to shop for foods with wisdom.

Three Breakfast Ideas

Day 1—Wake-Up Oats

1 cup of raw oats
1 quart of water or almond milk
1 or 2 pieces of papaya
2 dates (*optional*)
2 ounces raisins
½ cup mixed nuts* (*optional*)
Dash of nutmeg
Dash of cinnamon
1 banana ** (If you suffer from constipation avoid bananas)
Few pieces of dried apple or 2 slices of fresh apple

Combine all the ingredients.

Bring to a boil a quart of water or vanilla or carob soy milk.

Pour hot liquid over other ingredients.

Mix well and enjoy.

One can mix lecithin and powdered Brewer's yeast for more variety, or one can use other fruits. Experiment and create different tastes.

A quick, easy nutritious breakfast will fill you up and give you energy throughout the day.

Note: Dried fruit is a sweets substitute. It is the lesser of two evils. Otherwise, one would eat oats alone and that would be too bland for most people. Natural sugar can be used in moderation.

Choose your sweetener. Use one or two pieces of dried papaya, raisins or dates, or, either fresh apples or pears. Papaya aids digestion. Omit bananas to avoid constipation.

** Bananas should have spots on them so that, instead of being in their starchy state, which will cause you gas and constipation, they are in their natural sugar state.

* Soak overnight for easier digestion.

Day 2 —Fruit Breakfast

1 grapefruit diced

3-4 slices of pineapple

1 orange

½ cup cherries

½ cup grapes

Have a healthy fruit combination to start off your day.

Day 3 — Pick Me Up

1 cup of freshly prepared pineapple juice

1 cup of freshly prepared orange juice

1 tablespoon of Spirulina (*You can substitute chlorophyll or Heal Thyself Green Life Formula.*)

A delicious, powerful, health drink to start off your day.

Three Lunch/Dinner Ideas

Day 1 — Melange Supreme

1 or 2 eggplants (*melange*)
1 cup of water
1 or 2 sprigs of thyme
2 cloves of garlic
2 tablespoons of garlic oil
1 tablespoon grated diced ginger

Wash and cut eggplant into cubes.

Chop garlic and ginger; sauté in oil until brown.

Add eggplant, thyme, a cup of water and cook until eggplant is tender and completely mashed.

Add seasoning to taste or a pinch of cayenne pepper if one likes it hot.

Can be served over rice with vegetables and a salad.

Note: Always serve a smaller portion for your dinner meal.

Day 2 — Lentil Soup

1½ cups of lentils
1-2 potatoes and/or 1 cup of pumpkin
2 sprigs of thyme
2 cloves of garlic
1 piece of chopped ginger
1 onion
2-3 scallions
1 tablespoon of olive oil
Spike seasoning or any veggie seasoning

Wash lentils and put lentils in half a pot of water with garlic, ginger, thyme, oil and seasoning.

When lentils are halfway soft, wash potatoes and pumpkin.

Peel and cut into chunks: potatoes, green bananas and pumpkin.

Day 3-Trinidad Callaloo

16-20 dasheen or eddo leaves *(found in most Caribbean vegetable stores)*
2 packages of spinach or 2-3 bunches of fresh spinach
½ cup pumpkin
4 tablespoons of olive oil or any unsaturated oils
   (add to when dish has been prepared and removed from the fire)
2 blades of scallions
8-10 okras
1 large coconut or 2 tablespoons creamed coconut
1 green hot pepper
1 onion
1 sprig of thyme
½ pot of water

Wash leaves and break into small pieces.

Cut up okra.

Grate coconut, add 2 cups of hot water and extract coconut milk; or use 2 tablespoons of creamed coconut.

Place ingredients in pot (put in the hot pepper whole) and leave to boil until leaves are tender and okra seeds are pink.

Use a low fire. Swizzle or use a blender for a quick second.

Put mixture back into pot and simmer.

Add seasoning to taste.

Note: Do not blend in the hot pepper, the hot pepper is for flavoring. Put it back in when the callaloo is simmering.

This callaloo dish can be enjoyed as a soup by itself or one can incorporate with a variety of dishes to serve a fuller meal, e.g. steamed or boiled corn, brown rice, steamed or boiled plantains (green or yellow) or young green bananas, or a salad.

Tahoma Formula For Pregnant Women

Tahoma is a nurse/midwife who has performed home births over the years that I have known her. She has delivered hundreds of babies into the world in a loving home atmosphere throughout New York City. To extend her care to pregnant women, Tahoma is presenting here her # 2 Formula to make child-birth easier.

I. Acid Fruit Breakfast

Choices for cleansing of colds, sinuses and respiratory congestion.

> 1 grapefruit (diced)
> 3-4 slices of pineapples
> 1 orange (sliced)

II. Fruit Breakfast

> ½ cup cherries
> ½ cup strawberries
> ½ cup blueberries
> ½ cup raspberries

Have a healthy fruit combination to start off your day!

"MAMA AFUA'S" Children's Kitchen

Children's Food for Holistic Living

Vegetarian foods help prevent childhood illnesses.
Simple supper suggestions include:

- **Soyaburger on a whole wheat bun and sprouts;**
- **Soyafrank on whole wheat and sugarless mustard;**
- **Spinach or whole-wheat spaghetti with grated tofu and to-mato sauce with soya sauce for taste.**

Have a glass of vegetable juice 1-hour before each meal. Eat a large salad with every. Consume vegetable okra soup 1-2 times a week to maintain a cleansed colon.

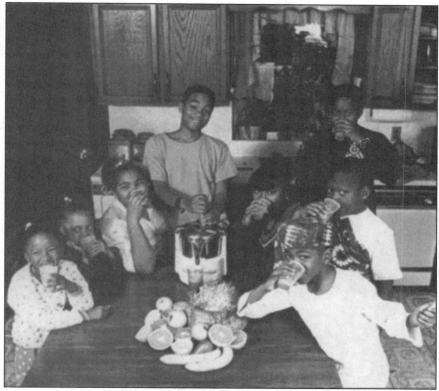

Children's Lunches

Monday   Tofu sandwich on sprouted whole wheat bread (tofu cake, 1 tablespoon unsalted mustard, tamari to taste; blend and spread on bread; top with lettuce or sprouts).

Tuesday   Vegetables in a pita pocket. Add lettuce, grated carrots, sprouts, and grated beets. (*Optional:* tahini butter or avocado spread.)

Wednesday   Raw almond or peanut butter on rice or sesame cakes or whole wheat bread.

Thursday   Vegetable soup in a Thermos jug with sea weed crackers.

Friday   Soy burger on whole-wheat bun with sugar-less and salt-less catsup.

In lunch box, add soymilk, *un*sweetened fruit juices or freshly pressed juices, 1-2 pieces of fruit, 1 ounce raw nuts (soak overnight for easier digestion). You also may add dried fruits in moderation.

Remember to toast all breads that are used.

If your child catches a cold, have him/her eat fruits for one or two days and avoid cooked food. Also give your child an herbal laxative after school, as well as one grapefruit each day s/he is ill.

Twelve

Breaking
Addiction
Naturally

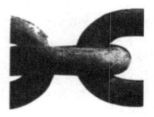

The root word for addictions is addict, which means to devote or give oneself habitually or compulsively; one awarded to another like a slave.

WHEN WE'RE ADDICTED to anything or to anyone, our lives are not our own. We may have good intentions, but we can't seem to follow through on our mission. Our hopes and dreams and high aspirations are put at bay because we can't or don't know how to diffuse the addiction. Addictions, all of them, just drain our energy force; leaving us less than who we are.

We, as human beings, are all addicted to something or to someone. An addictive state is when your right divine mind says "no," but a deep force within your body says "yes" to the almighty Addiction.

Toxic food has taken you in, once again, as you say, "All I need is one more taste," and so you proceed. You're going down. Then, your right, divine mind yells louder, 'cause you are beginning to feel the pain of the hard, cold addiction, and so you drink, rescue yourself quickly with your live juice and eat plenty of greens and soya foods as you hear positive empowering affirmations, pumping yourself back up again.

You're doing well for a few days, maybe even a few weeks. You have suppressed the urge. Then, challenge enters in, such as a canceled love date, a family feud, stress on the job, or, simply, someone else's bad attitude, and there you go again, down the dark, bleak avenue where addiction awaits you and willingly takes you in. Some say, "My addiction is not so bad, at least I'm not addicted to drugs or alcohol; I'm just addicted to food." Think again! Addiction to toxic food will cause a cancer to spread, a tumor to grow, blood pressure to rise and arthritis to eat up your bones and nerves. Ask yourself are any addictions safe?

Addictions come in many forms and fashions. Relationship blues of toxic lovers, mates and friends are only images of who and what we have been. So, we limit and/or end the toxic, abusive relationships. Then, time passes and we don't necessarily heal or cleanse that part of ourselves that attracted such a challenging mate or friend. Only this time, he or she has a different suit, cloth, drape, job or car. In truth, we did not take the necessary time and healing lessons that each relationship brings. So, we walk through the same pain once again. At first, the toxic relationship tastes good and is very pleasurable and stimulating. Then sooner or later naiveté, (lack of light, or) wickedness of our inner self, through the relationship, reveals itself. We are caught up in an endless cycle, for we are addicted to our old attitudes, needs, and desires; we got the relationship blues.

Cigarette toters, alcohol-drinkers, drug-addicts say, "This is my last 'hit' or 'smack.' Just one more time; after this time I won't do it again," until the next time and it happens again and again and again... So you shoot up, or snort up, booze up, or take one more puff and your visions and great plans go up in smoke. You gonna have to tie your addiction to a tree and wipe some herbs and bushes into it and begin to put your life in divine order.

You must believe that an addiction is an addiction, is an addiction! They really are one in the same. An addiction seems to numb the pain, numb your fears or suppress rage, when, in fact, the challenges of life become more acute as we are lead by our many conscious and unconscious addictions. Stop fighting for, supporting or defending your addiction. It's only purpose is to destroy you and those close to you.

Our addictive behaviors are passed down from one generation to the next. It begins in the womb. Children learn of toxic, addictive food via their mother's and father's consumption. The mother continues the food legacy of what her mother prepared in the kitchen, thereby, passing the toxic, addictive food down to the child. From kitchen to kitchen, over generations, the food that a woman consumes creates an energy field that attracts a mate, that reflects the woman, that brings forth the quality of the offspring one births.

In the event that the woman mates and conceives a child, the fetus grows from the combined food consciousness of the joint union of woman to man. The toxic food addiction established in the womb, and our DNA, develops a 'blue print' or 'black print' of toxicity from birth, childhood, teen life, to adulthood.

We continue the toxic or healthy food chain that our families offered to us as an extension of their love, their knowledge, or lack of. If the foods are toxic, ultimately, the addiction for these toxic foods must be broken for the renewal and resurrection of our body Temple via our restored kitchen Healing Laboratory.

Change your Karma for your survival, by flushing out your addiction through Nutritional Fasting and Natural Living. No longer weakened, but empower yourself and your entire family line, past, present, and future, by releasing every legal and illegal addiction, that this addictive society and world does or does not condone. Be steadfast and know that you have the power to overcome every ill, for you are bigger than any and every addiction.

Anti-Addiction Prayer and Affirmation

Today, I affirm that I am free of all addiction.

With my nature helpers, Herbal tonic, Live Green juice and Natural food and Healing Prayer and Affirmations spoken,

I am free of past pain, disappointments and hurts.

I claim Freedom from oppressors in the form of Drugs, Alcohol, Sugar, Flesh Foods, Junk Foods and Toxic Relationships.

I am more powerful than any and all addictions.

Right now, I take control of my life, I steer my ship to a safe, healthy harbor.

Today, I commit to give myself 21 days, 12 weeks, 365 days to begin the transforming process into the real me, one who is addiction-free!

Natural Living

The Road To Freedom

For all those who have been caught up in the web of a destructive life style of gloom and doom, who are locked in an illusion of reality, there is a salvation message for you.

The way to break your addiction is to detoxify your life by Natural Living and Live Juice Fasting with the Heal Thyself Principles. Consistently, through upholding and ingesting the tools of the Creator through air, fire, water and earth, by way of Nature, join the path of Purification to transmute your addiction into love, health and peace. The Freedom Call is beckoning you to reclaim your light and your victory.

For Crack, Cocaine or Potato Chip Lovers

For Cigarette smokers or Flesh eaters

For Sugar addicts or Starch consumers

For Greasy spoon eaters or Sex abusers

For Junk Food Indulgers or Soda Drinkers

There is hope for you.

Drug Addictions and The Statistics

Cocaine and Crack

In the New York City metropolitan area, DAWN figures for cocaine-involved deaths showed an increase beginning 1993. In 1993, the number increased 12 percent in 1 year to 815 deaths. Among ED patients in the first six months of 1995, males continue to dominate in the number of deaths. (71 percent). Blacks continue to represent the majority of cocaine abusers. The first half of 1995, however, saw an exceedingly large number of primary cocaine admissions.

The modes specified are smoking crack (about 72 percent of admissions) and inhaling or snorting cocaine (25 percent). The majority of primary cocaine admissions are males (60 percent), Blacks (65 percent). Those who were already in treatment amount to over two-thirds of those counted in the study. Many of those admitted did so, due to alcohol abuse.

Field researchers report that more young people are smoking marijuana joints or "blunt" cigars laced with crack. The street term for these joints or cigars is "woolies."

Heroin

DAWN figures for heroin-involved deaths in the New York City metropolitan area have shown a steady increase since 1994. Between 1990 and 1993, the number of deaths increased 42 percent, from 557 to 793. Heroine-involved ED mentions have also increased between 1990 and 1993, nearly tripling from 3,810 to 11,351.

Marijuana

Marijuana activity in New York City continues to evidence dramatic increases. The total number of marijuana ED mentions, projected from current sample of hospitals, had more than doubled in 1991, from 1,196 to 2,589. The estimate of marijuana mentions for the first six months of 1995 for the New York metropolitan area at 1,524 represents a rate of 18.0 per 100,000 population, nearly twice the national average of 10.3. In fact, the number nearly doubled between 1990 and 1994 from 1,662 to 3,294.

Psychoactive Prescription Drugs

Hospital emergencies and treatment admissions indicated that the non-medical use of psychoactive drugs is not a serious problem; however, the Street Studies Unit continues to report that alprazolam, amitriptyline, and hdyromorphone (Dilaudid) are readily available on the streets of New York City.

In addition, if you are a statistic, you can remove yourself from the list by taking on a life style of Purification & Rejuvenation.

Source: New York State Alcoholism and Substance Abuse Services (OASAS).

Drug Abuse Ongoing Crisis

Presently, the statistics have changed, but as of September 2001, there are still staggering numbers of people who are addicted to one or more dangerous, harmful and, sometimes, illegal substances.

In 1999, an estimated 14.8 million Americans were using an illicit drug, of that number 75 percent were using marijuana, while 43 percent during that same survey or an estimated 6.4 million Americans were using other illicit drugs, excluding and including those using marijuana and hashish. This is according to the United States Department of Health and Human Services, Substance Abuse and Mental Health Services Administration's website to be found at the following address: www.samhsa.gov/uas/nhsda/1999/chapter2.htm.

The survey reported that about 1.5 million people were current cocaine users, while about 413,000 represented current crack addicts. In addition, it found that 900,000 Americans were using hallucinogens and about 200,000 Americans were using heroin. While 75 percent of the drug users were also using or solely using marijuana, those who used marijuana solely accounted for 57 percent of those surveyed. Four million Americans used psychotherapeutic drugs, non-medically, representing 1.8 percent of the population, aged 12 and older, as in all of the survey cases.

It should be noted that there were no deaths from marijuana, according to the World Almanacs, Life Insurance Actuarial rates and the last 20 years of the United States Surgeon General's reports, as cited at the following website http://mojo.calyx.com/~umacrc/library/how_dangerous. However, illicit drug overdose (deliberate or accidental) caused 3,800 to 5,200 deaths, and alcohol use caused 150,000 deaths.

Sample Food Addictions

Eating until you're full and still you can't stop. Eating yourself to sleep. Eating to numb out your troubles and suppress emotional and psychological pain. Eating for fulfillment and still coming up empty. Eating because you can't have it; the thing, the person, the money, etc. Eating in this low vibrational manner is what's causing our lives to be stagnated and filled with grief.

Some people eat; then force themselves to throw it up. Eating and you're not hungry; eating misery away, eating in place of sex, eating for sex. Is what you're eating, eating away at your good, your peace, your joy?

Eating foods that you know are causing you bodily harm i.e. headaches, high blood pressure, asthma, obesity from such foods as fast foods, junk foods, flesh foods, sugar and salt, is destructive. We must purify out of our systems foods and non-foods that are non-nutritious, that cause bodily harm i.e. such as the previous foods mentioned. You can't seem to say no? Do you sneak and eat behind close doors and come up feeling guilty about what you ate.

If you want to stop overeating, but the food keeps calling you: Know that you are trapped into eating blues; you are addicted to a disorder of a legal drug called food.

Embrace this body of holistic works so the food addiction will be behind you.

The Voice of Relationship Addicts, to Toxic Food and other Vices

- I've got to have him or her, although I know deep down inside that she/he is no good for me—pass the chips.
- We have nothing in common; I don't even like him but the sex is good—pass the ice-cream.
- We've been together now for two years; I know he's married, but he promised to leave her for me—pass the rolls.
- She verbally abuses me, but I love her. He slapped me up, but I was asking for it. I can't leave him; he means well—give me some beer.
- This is the last time I'm going to forgive him for sleeping around; he said he's sorry and he won't do it again—pass the smoke.
- Yea, she puts me down all the time, makes me feel like nothing, but we have children together—I'll take a double serving of fried chicken wings.
- If you hit me one more time, I'm leaving—cut me a second slice of pound cake,

- If you find yourself making any of these statements or excuses for staying in a toxic union, then know that you are strung out and in an addictive, abusive relationship that will overtime distort you. Detox your life, your thoughts, your actions, your words, your diet, your home, your body Temple with the Heal Thyself Fasting and Natural principles. Maintain a holistic life style and overtime you will flush out the many levels of relationship blues.

One Path To Freedom

A devotee of the path of Heal Thyself has a miracle to share with us on his journey of addictive-free living and how he was able to heal himself naturally through wholistic living. Pay close attention. You will witness how even major addictions can be broken and how one overcame to the point of being an example and inspiration for others to heal themselves. Heru Pa-Ur Tehuti se Ptah is now a profound Heal Thyself teacher of fasting and Natural Living. He was so charged by his healing that he also became a Heal Thyself 'Soul Sweat' facilitator, and has guided thousands unto the path of purification. This is an example of a Lotus man; out of the mud of challenge came forth the lotus. This is the story of Pa-Ur's resurrection.

As a young man, Heru Pa-Ur Tehuti se Ptah started drinking alcohol, which we know is legal and accepted. Pa-Ur says "you really never know the effects of drinking until it is too late. Alcohol is lethal. It works slowly on destroying the system.

I never knew that I was addicted to alcohol. I drank alcohol almost every day. No one could tell me that I was addicted to alcohol. Most people who drink alcohol, drink at least once or twice a week or more. But, you could never tell them, they are alcoholics. Self-denial is at hand.

Then, I started smoking cigarettes. To me, this was the greatest of all my addictions. I called cigarettes *"nico-the-teen."* For it is the youngest of all the addictions. Smoking cigarettes was as normal as drinking was, because it was accepted and most people don't look at someone who smokes as weak, or dangerous, or an addict. Smoking and drinking are usually the first stages of addiction. Smoking and drinking are dangerous drugs, sanctioned by our government. For me, they opened doors to pot, cocaine, heroine, painkillers (prescription drugs), methadone and others. At one time, I was using and addicted to these drugs.

In 1986, I had a spinal operation. Upon my release from the hospital, I was prescribed 3,000 mg. of painkillers and muscle relaxers a day. The pain was still there so I added painkillers with codeine, vodka, wine, crack, and cocaine. I shot coke and heroine, and from time to time took methadone. In the year of 1991, I decided to save my life. This was not an easy task, but my desire to live, my desire to set a good example for my seven children and for others was a burning desire. Together with my beloved brother, Hru Ankh Ra Sen-Ur Semahj se Ptah and Queen Afua Mut Nebt-Het, I started a process of "Liberation through Purification." A painstaking task of reclaiming myself.

* * *

My first step was to stop drinking, for drinking was the source, and the energizing factor in my addictions. I didn't slow down. I stopped. It was very painful to stop. I began eating lots of fruits and drinking a lot of water. I also began drinking a lot of green vegetable juice. My constant thought was to save my life. I knew I was dying; there was no doubt in my mind. My body was closing down. The entire left side of my body seemed to be blocked. My body was preparing for a stroke or a heart attack. The pain was severe and the drugs, that I was using to stop the pain, were creating more and more pain. But, I was determined to save my life. This poem may explain:

Just In Time

Just In Time!
Just in the 'nick of Time'
My life was saved
I was moving about doing crazy things
and hurtful things
and just when My life had run into a place

where death was holding a meeting
and invited me in
My life was spared
Just In the 'nick of Time!'

Weakness could no longer rule,
for strength insisted on, driving my body, mind and spirit.
Just in the 'nick of time'

My precious life was almost lost. . .
I had almost lost the gift,
but just in the 'nick of time'
I was able to rise from the grave of pain and weakness

I give praise and thanks for the gift of strength
Praise the Divine,
oh Praise the Divine
The Great Protector who allows us to make mistakes
 and also Blesses us to Resurrect Ourselves,
I give praise and thanks
for being able to Recover
Just in the 'nick of Time!'

Steps to Healing

Before taking on the Heal Thyself 21-Day Fast on live foods, I had to detoxify my body. My beloved brother Hru Ankh Ra Sen-Ur Semahj se Ptah started taking me to the bath house to do deep sweating, for several hours at a time. This was a helping factor, for I began to clean the largest organ of the body, the skin. This process took place every week with clay packs, Breath of Spring, and Heal Thyself Formula 1 and Formula 2. Within the first month, I had won the battle against alcohol, prescription drugs, cocaine, crack and heroin; one day at a time. But, my body was weak and the pain wasn't going anywhere. Sometimes, I wanted to go back to those things. But my desire to live was greater. In simple but strong words, "I wanted to live."

I was still smoking cigarettes and pot, but I knew I had to come all the way back and that the work could be difficult. I started praying and praying hard, asking for strength. I was told that the strength that I needed was inside of me. It was standing right there next to my weaknesses. On the second month of my journey, I stopped eating meat. That was not hard, for I still had chicken, goat and fish. Four months went by and I began to get stronger in my healing. I was juicing every day and going to the bathhouse once or twice a week. Also the gift of carving wood was very helpful to me. It allowed me to really see and feel the process of transformation. As I began carving wood, I was also cutting away from my life things that were harmful to me.

One night, I decided to take on "nico-the-teen." So, I took the cigarettes and placed them on my dresser and spoke to them saying, "Tonight is the night!"

Before going to bed, I would smoke a cigarette, drink some water and go to sleep. But, this night I decided to take on my greatest addiction. I spoke to it because it was real. I told "nico-the-teen" that I was willing to throw up, pee on myself, and even doo-doo on myself, but I was not going to smoke; and I did not. I tossed and turned some of the night; I almost gave up. I tried to comfort myself by saying, "I will stop tomorrow," but I was deep in the battle. I woke in the morning victorious!

My first week was my greatest achievement of my journey. Everything else began to come easy. After eight months, I decided, with the help and blessings of the heavyweight champion of purification, Queen Afua Mut Nebt-Het, that I would accept the gift of the Heal Thyself 21-Day Fast. This program was the foundation to my really seeing clearer. After that, everything became a little easier. Formula 2 Master Herbal Formula was a day-to-day helper in keeping the urges of addiction from returning. My first year was glorious. The beginning of the second year, I left chicken alone, and six months later fish. Then, I heard a calling inside of me, saying, "What are you going to do for me?" I asked, "Who's that speaking to me?" The voice said, "I am the lungs, the keeper of the breath." The lungs stated that I was doing such a wonderful job healing the rest of the Temple and wanted to know how come I was not looking out for them. I stated that I had already stopped smoking cigarettes and they said, "Yes, but you are still smoking pot." I answered back justifying my actions, "Pot is an herb from the earth." The lungs said, "You are right, but I can only filter oxygen and not smoke." So, I made a promise to my lungs to stop smoking pot. Spring of that year, I was once again victorious!

I would like to give praise and thanks to the wonderful; and powerful Creator NTR, for blessing me to be on this journey for more than 10 years and for being victorious over my addictions.

* * *

Today, years later Heru Pa-Ur Tehuti se Ptah is a true shining example of an upright, purified, Lotus man who has inspired numerous sisters and brothers to begin breaking their addictions. He has shown them how to free themselves by naturally Healing Thyself. Pa-Ur is now a certified Heal Thyself Fasting Instructor. May the Creator continue to watch over Pa-Ur and give him continued peace and healing.

* * *

I've included the following poem as inspiration to those striving to overcome addictions. I admire Snt Tehuti and others like her who from her beginnings, on the Path of Purification, was committed to healing herself systematically, breaking her addiction, which had accelerated over her lifetime. Her graduation of body-mind, spiritual ascension is expressed in this poem. Keep this thought close to your heart that like Pa-Ur, Snt Tehuti and others, we all have the power to free ourselves of every addiction.

If I Can, You Can, It's All Up to You

by Snt Tehuti

I had some interesting things happen in my days
I allowed so much to happen in so many ways
I allowed anxiety, frustration, and hardheadedness to overrule
I had so much to learn and I wasn't going to get it at school
It all started one day to many months and years after that
The motive of my addictions stemmed from a lack of something and that's a fact

I developed a habit and held on to past stuff
Constantly thinking why, how come, until I shouted enough!
I couldn't function unless there was much drama
My addictions were many results of my own karma
Repetitive, negative behavior and events were the stage
And, in my heart, I was deeply enraged
At the results of my not paying attention to the signs that were there
Oh, did I forget to mention, that at the time, I really didn't care
Those addictive relationships kind of helped me escape
To an unknown reality that couldn't even be taped
Because those relationships that I didn't investigate
Caused me to get deeper and deeper until it was almost too late
My allergies, cramps, and depression made me feel so bad
The low-vibrational people, foods, and drinks caused me to feel sad
For I wined and I wined and I felt so unfulfilled
I kept saying "I'm gonna try" until I changed it by saying "I will"
I was faxed information about a center called Heal Thyself.
I signed up for the 21-Day Fasting Program to improve my health
I prepared the formulas, live foods, juices. So much work I had to do
Internal cleansing, clay packs, salt baths, meditation—
this was all new. I fasted for my earth years, my sins and my life to be
made anew
And don't forget Creator, please save me from my addictions, too!
The lessons I learned was to maintain a light and clean heart
To prevent addictions from turning into dis-ease is a start
To me, it was a blessing and there's much more I could say
The Creator was in the plan and guided me on my way
I continue to work to break my addictions and bring forth my good
qualities to the surface.
I healed myself; to be made a new
as I prayed to the Creator to save me from my addictive state of being.
For if I can, you can, it's all up to you.

Anti-Addiction Natural Life Style Diet

(12 weeks to 365 Days)

The Heal Thyself Life Style Diet will purify and restore the blood. The blood stream cleanses itself naturally if not poisoned by toxic, fast or processed foods being eaten. If we have polluted our bloodstream through toxic consumption, then we can help to purify and rejuvenate the blood with red foods, such as cranberry juice, beets and berries. The most important key to remember when breaking any addiction is that you must purify the blood. As you purify the blood so you purify your body Temple; so here goes.

Perform: The Heal Thyself Purification Prayer at sunrise to establish your day and again at sunset to give thanks for successfully winning the war over your addiction for just one more day. Even if you have been challenged, give thanks for another opportunity to try to do better again this time. I have been a witness to thousands over the years that have overcome many levels of addictions. I know that you can overcome. Come on, I will show you how to reclaim your ticket to freedom. Let's begin our day.

It's Pre-Breakfast Time:

Blend together:

        Juice of lemons

        2 cloves of garlic

        ¼ cup of Aloe Vera

        12 ounces warm distilled water

Breakfast:

(Liquid Breakfast)

        8-12 ounces fresh fruit juice (bitter fruit juices are the best)

        Unsweetened Cranberry or Grapefruit with distilled water

        Drink 8-12 ounces of water with or after juice. Add 1-2 teaspoon of Heal Thyself Green Life Formula

(Solid Breakfast)

2-3 pieces of fruits in proper food combination only
Acid fruit i.e. grapefruit, oranges, pineapple
Sub-acid fruit: pears, apples, berries, etc.
Melon i.e. cantaloupe, honeydew, watermelon
1 to 2 teaspoons of Heal Thyself Green Life

Don't Miss Lunch (Maintain your balance)

(Liquid Lunch)

12-16 ounces of Green Vegetable Juice with 1-2 teaspoons of Green Life Formula
1-2 hours later enjoy your solid lunch

(Solid Lunch)

Large salad (*add kelp or dulse* as a nutritional seasoning) steamed vegetables (*3-4 minutes.*)

Vegetable protein (TVP, peas, beans, sprouts, raw soaked seeds/nuts), baked unshelled fish as a transitional animal protein, 1-3 times a week, if not ready to be a complete vegetarian yet! I choose 1 protein per meal.

Beware of all soya products that contain eggs. If you consume eggs in any form, you are not practicing a vegetarian diet.

Choose 1 complex carbohydrate per meal i.e. couscous, tabouli, bulgar, millet.

Complex carbohydrates should be eaten once a day only in the mid-day to avoid constipation.

The Sun is Going Down. Let's Get Our
Dinner:

Repeat Lunch Menu

Follow Recipes in *The Heal Thyself Natural Living Cookbook* or *Kitchen Power* video for a variety of food options.

Note: Anyone interested in eating at a healthy vegetarian restaurant needs to check in their yellow pages, *Vegetarian Times* magazine, local health food stores, food co-ops and yoga and dance schools for guidance on restaurant locations in your area. If there are none in your community, you may decide to learn how to prepare vegetarian food and open your own restaurant as a service to the community.

Take the following nutritional supplements to rejuvenate your body Temple with freshly pressed vegetable or fruit juice for extreme additions.

2-4 tablespoons Spirulina

50-100 mg. Vitamin B Complex

1000 mg. Vitamin C

1-2 tablespoons of granulated Lecithin

(Take 3 times a day.)

1-2 ounces Fresh Wheatgrass

12-16 ounces of distilled water 3-7 times a week for a Master detox

For gentle detoxing, take Wheatgrass juice in the following way. Start with 1 ounce daily for 1 week. Increase to 2 ounces daily in the second week. After 2 weeks increase up to 4 ounces daily. For this amount, it's better to learn to grow your own wheatgrass at home so that you'll be able to juice it fresh and have larger quantities at an affordable cost. Or, simply buy fresh wheatgrass from a health food store.

As a starter, you can use the Heal Thyself Green Life Formula I 1-2 times for 3 or 4 days.

Green Vegetable Juice for a Natural High (1-2 times a day.)

> 4-8 ounces Dark Green juice i.e kale, spinach, broccoli, celery, parsley, etc.
>
> ½-1 Beet
>
> 1 Turnip
>
> 2 Scallions
>
> 2 Radishes
>
> *¼ cup of ginger-may be added to fruit or vegetable juices three times a week (Optional, but advisable.).

Herbal Laxative

> 3-4 tablets of casagrada sagrada at night with water for 21 days with warm distilled water (12-16 ounces).
>
> Drink bitters or Heal Thyself Master Herbal as often as possible to detoxify the body Temple of poisons particularly if cravings set in. This will help you to wash the craving away.

Music Healing

If you are a music lover, it is helpful to use music for healing, such as a string instrument, guitar, piano, harp, or zither. A wind instrument such as the flute or percussion instruments such as the tempora are also helpful. Perhaps, you would like to explore making your own healing music with thumb pianos, African xylophones and other instruments. All these sounds can elevate your mind and spirit. Avoid harsh, staccato, or loud music. Turn off your television for 21 Days and get your thoughts back and flush some of the radiation out of your body Temple and environment.

Meditation

Work with a Meditation Teacher (Guide) to help you to develop innate peace and emotional stability. Once you learn to meditate as a wonderful form of stress management, practice meditation at home starting with 5 minutes, building up to as much as 30 minutes daily. Meditation can be done with or without music. Learn to listen to the still, quiet music of your soul. Read *Sacred Woman: A Guide To*

Healing the Feminine Body, Mind and Spirit; it's filled with meditation exercises. MAAT meditation is the one I recommend to balance out your inner being. This MAAT meditation can support both women and men.

Prepare **Master Herbal Formula #2**

> Prepare your own or purchase Heal Thyself Master Herbal Formula and break your addictions naturally.
>
> 3-5 tablespoons to 5-6 cups of water.
>
> Steep overnight; strain in the morning and drink before 1:00 p.m.

Hot water Salt

Bath for deep relaxation and detoxification (Take 3-7 baths per week.)

> 2-4 pounds of Epsom salt
>
> Soak 30 minutes to one hour. Hot shower after bath.
>
> Self-massage body from head to toe.
>
> Drink 1 quart of water while in the tub. (Add 1 tablespoon of spirulina to rejuvenate or 4 teaspoon of goldenseal to water to detox.)

Clay Pack

> Apply over liver each night a clay pack with gauze; take a hot shower in morning to wash the clay pack off.
>
> Apply Rejuvenation Clay over any areas in the body that are lacking circulation and to draw out toxins that have accumulated from the addiction.

Sweat Bath, Sauna, Steam bath, Russian or Turkish Bath should be done 1-3 times a week for 1-2 hours at a time. Shower in between the sweat as the layers of poisons are released through the skin. While in the tub, drink distilled water, bitter herbal tea, or lime water. Massage entire body from foot to head.

Exercise: Work It Out Through Exercise for 15-30 minutes or more, daily or twice a week i.e., power walking (especially in a natural setting when possible for fresh air), biking, jogging, swimming, dancing, aerobics, etc. In all, perform deep breathing throughout sessions; you'll feel revitalized within a short time. Perform Fire-Breath 100-300 times a day.

Herbal Relaxer

When feeling stressed out or pressured, or tearful, take a cup of nature in a tonic:

* 1 teaspoon Valerian
* 2-4 teaspoon Chamomile
* 2-4 teaspoon Hops

Boil 4-6 cups of water; turn off pot. Then add above herbal formula; steep overnight drain and drink by midday. Take this formula for at least 21 days before going to bed.

Beware! The Company You Keep Reflects Who You Are!

The quality of the company you keep will determine your success in breaking or not breaking your addictive patterns. Learn to enjoy your own company or the company of those who are striving to move in the same direction of wellness, as yourself. After about 12 weeks to a year of strengthening and detoxing yourself, you may go back and help others who are in trouble and who are ready to experience a wholistic transformation and grow out of their addiction. After a season of 365 days of consistent cleansing and rejuvenation, you would have improved enough to reach back to your past and aid someone else who is in need of healing. But, go forth and Heal Thyself first; be a mighty example. Keeping in mind that some relationships you need not enter again; trust your spirit to guide. Travel with a light heart; know that we learn much from each relationship that we have been drawn to. Be brave; let go of toxic patterns. Otherwise, you may go under with them and find yourself recycling addictive behavior once again.

Body Work

As you take on this Natural Life Style and become more committed in reclaiming your life, it is advisable to connect with an acupuncturist, such as can be found at the Lincoln Hospital/Substance Abuse clinic in the Bronx, New York.

Receive deep tissue massages 1-3 times a week, or as often as possible to increase circulation and to restore the blood and to drain mucus and congestion and stress out of the lymphatic system. (Such massage must be given by a professional masseuse/masseur, or a loving friend.) As you begin your bodywork, see your addictions leaving your life. As you heal, see the underlying reasons for your addiction as you bless your addiction away.

Wellness Progress Chart

Once you have been off the addiction for 21-days or more, please record the date of your accomplishment. That is the turning point of your recovery as you ascend on the road to freedom from your particular addiction. Moving from 21 to 42 days to 63 days to 84 days and, eventually to 365-days of uninterrupted purification would have you reach a maximum level of liberation.

Check off every 21-Days of Your Success over the said addiction.

➔ one year to self-mastery

Check off type of Addiction		21	42	63	84	281	365
Please check off the date of your success							
CHECK OFF ADDICTION							
DRUGS							
crack/cocaine/heroin/marijuana							
prescription medication							
alcohol							
tobacco							
TOXIC FOOD							
flesh food							
pork, beef, chicken, fish (circle)							
sugar (brown or white)							
coffee							
dairy							
starch							
JUNK FOODS							
chips, candy, soda (circle)							
TOXIC RELATIONSHIP							
toxic mate							
toxic friend							
toxic sexual union							
other:							

Comments: Write in comments. If you have a tape, indicate what happens to challenge you, then return to your purification as you detox from your addiction.

Every seasonal change, you go through a deeper level of cleansing so record the addiction that leaves out with the change of the season.

In column one, record the addiction.

In column two, record the number of days without the toxic substance.

Support Group

Develop a group of those who have common wellness goals and work collectively over a 21-Day, 12-Week, 365-Day period. Start simple with the group 1-Day Fasting Shut-In and grow into your wellness with new and higher reflections.

Be patient and gentle with yourself as you rise and whatever happens hold no guilt!

It's important when cleansing not to harbor feelings of guilt or hide from yourself for shame. Remember "Every Lesson Is A Blessing!" If you happen to act on your addiction in the midst of cleansing, worry not. For each day of your wellness, the cravings will become less and less. So commit to purify. Affirm I am and I will be victorious. Bless Yourself and pick yourself up sweetly. The next meal eat and drink from the nectar of the Most High. As you envision your journey of 21 Days, 84 Days and, finally, 365 Days from now, you would have built a body Temple of Pure Divine Light, so be patient, but diligent, devoted and committed to your 100% wellness.

Note for Helpers

Mothers, Fathers, Husbands, Wives,

Lovers, Relatives and Friends:

When striving to detox a loved one, if they are in need and you are able, assist them by preparing their tonics and baths for 21 Days or more. Pray and meditate with them if time permits.

From your efforts, they will receive great empowerment and so, will be inspired to carry the torch of light for themselves, from this point forward, because you gave them a helping hand.

If the person in need is at a far distance; a phone call a few times a week, may be all they need for inspiration to move forward and break the addiction(s).

While you're helping them to break their addiction, work your own, for every human being has an addiction or two; it's all a part of living and functioning in the mundane plan.

Thirteen

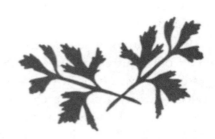

Nature Cures

A Personal Interview with Mother Lucille Law and other Folk Healers

THE SPIRIT OF Mother Lucille Law, mother of WWRL Radio personality Bob Law, resides in all our families. Think back! Remember an aunt, a grandmother, an uncle, a grandfather or an elder of the family, community, village or compound who carried within them the knowledge of the plants: like that of George Washington Carver who talked to plants and Harriet Tubman who used herbs to heal us as we traveled the underground railroad.

Talk to and study from the elders; they have the keys to our wellness then and now. Remember the ancient ones of the Nile Valley, Imhotep, the father of ancient and modern medicines and Ast (Isis), the first mother of healing, who was astute in nature cures. The Healers! They are calling us to continue the work to preserve all the generations! The folk healers speak; dwell in us.

I had the privilege of meeting Mother Lucille Law, at my Brooklyn center years before her departure into the council of the ancestors. Mother Law shared her personal experience of being raised with natural remedies when she was a young girl.

"In the springtime when we children needed cleaning out, my father would make the boys go up in the pine trees to get pine cones.

My father would put all the hearts of those pine cones in a big pot and pour water over them, steam them and make a tea, adding our homemade syrup as sweetener. We had to take this tea for three nights straight and that cleaned us out. As a result of this, we didn't come down with pneumonia, even though we were running around barefoot and kicking up in the cold and what not. Nothing happened to us.

"Then, my mother would sometimes call to us and say, 'Go out in the field or out in the woods; I need some kind of root.' I can't even think of some of the roots now, but I do remember a couple of the names of the roots. She would send us out to pick the 'little plants,' as she would describe them to us and we listened very well. She would explain 'only the leaves that are like that,' or 'the flowers that are like this.' We would go out into the woods and come back with all kinds of little weeds and herbs. We would pull them up by the roots. She would look at them and pick out what she needed to make "*nip tea*" for the baby. The baby suffered with teething. She would take some of the other things and make some kind of tea for us. That was the way it was. Whatever that was, she never told us. She would just say, 'Come and drink this down,' whatever it was. All we knew was that we got better.

"There was a tea that she would make the girls take when their period was a little slow. She would give us pennyroyal tea. I remember when I went to her. I said, 'Mother Bryant, my period is acting up. It looks muddy or something.' She said, 'Nothing is wrong with you, but you caught cold. Go to the store and buy some pennyroyal.' I went and bought the pennyroyal, made the tea and it cleaned me out. My period came along normally."

"I came down with diphtheria. I was the only child in the family that had ever been laid up sick. Nobody was sick...and I caught diphtheria from my sister for she had attended a funeral or something where there was the germ. I was so sick with fever. I could see my chin. It was swollen all the way out. My father went out in the yard and got something that he called mullein and brought these big leaves into the house. He put them in a container with cold water. As fast as he put a leaf on my throat, it dried up. In fact, it would turn brown because my fever was so high. He stood by my bed, and, continually, put the leaves on my throat to break the fever. And you know what? He broke the fever with that herb."

"At that time, we would talk to the mothers at the Church. They would tell us what to do and we would get along 'awright.' I was at the Church for a long time. I was saved when I was a teenager. There was so much I didn't know that I had to talk to the mothers about."

Q: Were there any men, at that time, that you knew who had that same wisdom?

A: I think so. You see, my father had the wisdom about that pine tree and there were other things that he would do. They used to give us black draught. I don't know if they gave it to the younger children. There was a time when they put sulfur in shoes. Now, why, I don't know, but all of us had to wear sulfur in our shoes. After awhile, when the shoes got dirty or whatever, they would put more sulfur in our shoes. We had to wear the shoes with sulfur until they wore out. When we got another pair the same was repeated.

Q: During cleaning time, were there any specific things you had to do?

A: You mean for our bodies? We got that *pine top tea* in the beginning of the spring. The pine top tea cleaned us out in the spring.

* * *

Mother Law's son, Bob Law, remembers his mother's knowledge and use of natural cures.

"My brother and I were cutting wood and my brother split his foot wide open between the big toe. When Mama ran out, the blood was shooting out. The people wore long aprons, you know, (the mothers did) and she ran out and shouted, 'Bring some towels; bring some rags.' She jumped down on the ground on the boy's foot and she cupped it together and said, '*Go get me some spider web and get some soot out of the chimney.*' They were the only two things she called for and one of us ran to the chimney and the rest of us went to get the spider webs. Mother took the soot and put it right in that wide open cut that was bleeding. She took that spider web and put it right on top of the soot. She closed it altogether. We tore her apron and she bound the foot. She then put it in bags (what we call *croaker bags* or sack bags). She took that croaker sack, bound that boy's foot up, wiped it, and fixed it real well. She put him in a buggy with a horse and sent him to the doctor by himself. I'm not sure, at all, what the doctor did, but he did give my brother some stitches. He probably cleaned out all the stuff that my mother put in there, but she had stopped the bleeding. That stuff was to stop the bleeding and she stopped it. My brother would have bled to death. My mother saved his life."

* * *

During the days when Mother Law was a child and we, as a people, healed ourselves with nature cures, there were no doctors available to us. Thus, we followed Divine Laws for healing ourselves — the laws that the Creator gave us "To Be Ye Perfect."

We delivered our babies at home with the midwives or the "mothers of the church." Mothers were natural, then. They didn't use bottled milk from cows or goats, or formula manufactured in factories.

When we got fevers, female problems, aches and pain, or whatever the disease was, we used herbs that grew in the fields, mud from the earth, water from the stream and pot liquid from the greens to heal ourselves, to save ourselves. We were medically independent then; we were powerful, then and drug-free. We took care of each others' children and made them respect their elders at all costs. We kept our marriages and families together even when it was a modernized form of slavery because of the American enslavement. In the past, Black women ignored fathers and uncles raping daughters repeatedly, just to keep families together—women still do that today.

We had our babies at home. We had to be self-reliant in order to survive in business, in food production and labor. We could not have a family, even if in wounded states, imbalanced, we stood together to build our economics, our farms, our spirit that was destroyed from the years, eight to twelve generations of lost family.

If we are to regain the strength our elders had, we must return to the old ways, our traditional ways, the traditions of wholistic health that historically began in the Nile Valley of Khamit, and embrace natural healing.

We also have an array of new health products, herbs, vegetables, and oils such as olive, castor and almond to use.

We must love and respect our Afrikan *bush doctors* [herbalists], our midwives, our spiritualists, and our healers. We are truly equipped to heal ourselves. The purpose of *Heal Thyself* and *Sacred Woman* is to Heal your inner members, which causes a healing within your family, and create a family inspired to wholeness and oneness with the Divine. *As it was in the beginning, so shall it be in the end.* I thank Mother Lucille Law for sharing her experiences with us and reminding us of our ability to "Heal Thyself."

P.S. Mother Lucille Law passed soon after this interview. She was attended by seven ministers who conferred on her the title of Saint. It was, indeed, an honor to have been graced by her presence.

• • •

Cleansing is an Afrikan tradition that was carried over to the Caribbean Islands and the southern part of the United States. In most families, there was a healer who gathered the children, lined them up and gave them a bush tea or herb tea to purge them weekly or monthly. These healers, in most cases, helped to keep the children and adults free of disease.

While living in rural areas closer to nature, we ate pots of greens and drank bush tea. However, since migrating to the cities, we have been eating "fast food" and not getting much exercise, if any at all. Because we live less as collective family units, more diseases have been able to enter our bodies.

Natural Healing Is Not New To Many of the Folks in the Hills of Jamaica

It is our Divine right to heal ourselves. Paulette Herron was born and raised in Jamaica. She is the wife of a Rastafarian and the mother of three children. While I was in Jamaica, I had a brief interview with Sister Paulette. She shared with me knowledge about some of the herbs common to the Caribbean Islands. Many of these herbs cannot be obtained in health food stores, although they grow wild in the fields of the Caribbean. Here are some of the herbs, Sister Paulette shared with me.

- Fever grass -   for fevers
- Dandelion -   for colds
- Ram goat regular - for colds
- Donkey weed -   for colds
- Scorn the Earth - to strengthen a weak body

For swelling from a wasp's sting, mix three of any different kinds of tea leaves and rub on itchy, swelling area to relieve discomfort. Any three teas... what a miracle!

- For worms in children — soursop leaves
- Nervous breakdown — boil young Coconut with Strong Back Root and Irish Moss from the sea.

Peline is a young, hard-working, vegetarian man, born and raised in the hills of Jamaica, who freely shared some of the herbal knowledge that he was born into.

- *Strong Back Root* — to eliminate weakness and pain and "for men who are of no use to their women," as quoted.
- *Aloe* — for a blood wash-out.
- *Okra* — for fast delivery. (The mother of his son delivered her baby in 12 hours after labor began. She ate fresh okra from Peline's father's garden throughout her pregnancy). "The baby just slipped out at the appointed hour."
- *Thyme* — for easy birth.
- *Cerasee* — used for cleaning the colon (relieving constipation); for stomach pain and colds.
- *Dry Coconut* — to clean out your insides.

When in the Caribbean, Haiti, Afrika or Brazil, I always plan to visit the local "bush" doctor for natural healing direction and further information.

Nature Cures for Common Health Challenges

Clay

In the beginning God gave to every people a cup of clay and from this cup they drank their life.

Proverbs of Digger Indians

Clay is a "body food" that is nutritious. It stimulates, detoxifies and transforms the skin. It's a body food because it gives nourishment to the body internally and externally. Apply it with gauze to draw out poisons and to put minerals into an organ through the pores of the skin. According to the National Center of Scientific Research, clay contains: oxides and the chemical elements of silica, titanium, aluminum, iron, calcium, magnesium, sodium and potassium. From page 30 in the *Essene Gospel of Peace* on clay, we have the following:

I tell you truly, your bones will be healed. Be not discouraged, but seek for cure nigh the healer of bones, the angel of earth. For thence were your bones taken and thither will they return. And the knots of your bones will varnish away, and they will be straightened, and all your pains will disappear.

Queen Afua's Rejuvenating Clay

The Clay formula came together overtime. I healed myself naturally for seven years before I birthed and raised my three children.

I knew, early on, that I had to know as much as possible about natural living, which included knowing various nature cures if I was going to be a responsible Nature Mother, be their Nature Doctor, and raise my children drug, junk and toxic food free.

I began using clay before my daughter, Sherease's second birthday. At age 5, she fell off her bike and limped into the house, screaming as loud as she could, with what appeared to be a sprained arm and a swollen leg. I ran into the kitchen, pulled out the powdered clay and mixed it in a bowl with water, comfrey herb and other herbs. I mixed them into a compound, and with a wooden spoon, placed the clay on a gauze and wrapped her leg with the clay poultice.

I prepared her fresh, vegetable juice with spirulina, a seaweed algae, to help her to knit internally and to calm her nerves. After about 5-10 minutes, she stopped crying; I laid her upon her bed, kissed her forehead and allowed her to rest.

Sherease awoke about four hours later and started moving about like nothing happened. I gently showered off the clay pack. The swelling was down and the pain arrested. We winked at each other and broke into a smile.

That was my first time experiencing the miracle of clay. I successfully used clay throughout the years on myself, my children, my family, friends and clients.

Thirteen years ago, a client friend and astute businessman implored me to package and market my formula because he, too, was a recipient of the miracles of clay and he felt many people would embrace the rejuvenating qualities of clay.

Contents: green organic clay, red clover, comfrey and chaparral herbs, purified/distilled water and a touch of peppermint and eucalyptus oil.

Suggested uses:

Beauty Facial: to remove pimples, toxic lines and blackheads. Apply clay. Leave on for 30-45 minutes. Apply cucumber slices to eyes to decrease swelling. During this time lie at a 45⁰ angle. When clay drys wash face upward toward eyes with water or take a shower. Dry face, apply gel from aloe vera plant or use an aloe gel product from a health food store. Take 2 tablespoons of gel from aloe plant and combine with warm water and the juice of a lemon or lime, now drink, for true beautiful skin comes from within.

Draws out aches and pains:
Apply clay with gauze overnight. Remove by taking a warm shower in the morning.

Knits Bones: Apply with a gauze. Leave on overnight for best results. Shower off in the morning. Stay away from all sugar.

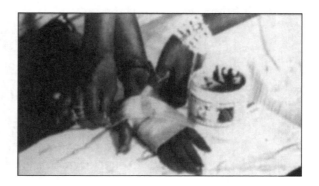

Strengthens scalp and hair:

> Massage aloe in scalp after drying wet hair. Apply clay into scalp and hair for at least 2 hours, then wash with Dr. Bronner's peppermint soap or black soap. Then massage *Queen Afua's Aloe Mist* or vitamin E oil into scalp.

Relieves Female Disorders:

> Use gauze or cotton swab to insert clay into vagina for 2-4 hours. Take a hot shower over the pelvic area after the clay has dried.

Whitens teeth and removes plaque:

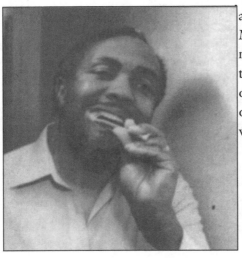

> Clay rejuvenates your mouth and prevents bleeding gums. Massage on gums or brush with non-abrasive toothbrush; allow to rest on gums for 1 hour with or without cotton. Then rinse out mouth with a cup of warm water and a pinch of sea salt.

Draws and cleanses body growth:

> Apply with gauze for 1 to 3 hours, or better, overnight.

Draws toxins from boils:

> Apply with gauze 1 teaspoon of clay and apply over boil overnight and shower in the morning. Air dry and cover with aloe gel during the day.

For full body cleaning:

> Shower with hot and cold water until totally cleansed, then apply clay over entire body. This procedure will remove dead skin, revitalize and refresh your skin and

cleanse clogged pores, so your skin can breathe.

For best results, while using Rejuvenation Clay, eat fresh fruits, vegetables, and drink *live juices and herb teas*. No sugar, dairy or fried foods. And take enemas or colonics at least 1-3 times a month during use of clay.

Internal Clay Tonic:

Take 1 teaspoon of clay and stir into 8 to 16 ounces of water and drink down every other day for detoxing your body Temple.

The Heal Thyself Self-Help Nutritional Program can aid in preventing or aiding the rejuvenation of the body Temple to build one's immune system to fight against many dis-eases.

Self-Help Nutritional Formula

You have choices, either consume the Heal Thyself Green Life Formula, which contains vegetarian calcium and vegetarian protein, B-Complex, Vitamin E, lecithin and psyllium husk. Take Green Life 3 times a day with vegetable or fruit juice, or create your own formula by combining the following vitamins and minerals below.

1-2 tablespoons powdered Spirulina

1-2 tablespoons powdered Wheatgrass

Contains vegetarian calcium and vegetarian protein and other mineral and vitamins.

25-50 mg. of Vitamin B to prevent stress. Protects hair, nerves and skin.

500-1,000 mg. of Vitamin C to help fight against bacteria, i.e. colds, sinuses, fever.

1 tablespoon granulated lecithin to decongest your arteries and to rejuvenate the brain cells.

1,000 mg. of calcium 1-2 times a day (If you suffer from arthritis and/or tooth decay.)

400 mg. of Vitamin E for oxygen and rejuvenation, to speed wellness, to clean the arteries, act as a brain food, and improve memory. Take once a day.

Add nutrients to the green vegetable juices or fruit juices.

Common Health Challenges

Daily Nature Cure Affirmation

As you drink your tonics, take your nutrients or bathe in a soothing bath, Affirm:

I am the likeness and image of the Most High; therefore, dis-ease is to be no more.

I will keep cleansing and detoxing until my body Temple reflects the pure light of my Maker.

Heal Thyself Formulas I, II and III can be applied to all health blockages listed. Meditation, affirmation, prayer and moderate exercises should accompany the healing for full recovery.

In preparing your herb tonics, add 3-4 teaspoons to 3-4 cups of warm water.

Steep 4 hours or overnight for a potent tonic.

Addiction to Drugs/Cigarettes

Herbs: Calamus root, alfalfa, dandelion, rosehips.

Nutrients: 1 to 4 ounces of spirulina daily

1000 mg. Vitamin C

50 mg. Vitamin B-Complex

Juices: Beets, wheatgrass, dark green veggies

Other: Clay pack over your liver

Acquired Immune Deficiency Syndrome (AIDS)

Herbs: Dandelion, red clover, alfalfa, goldenseal (take 4 teaspoons) for 14 days. Add powder to herbal tonics.

Juices: Beets, green leafy vegetables, scallions

Baths: 4-8 pounds of Epsom salts. (Warm water bath only if you have high blood pressure.) Add an additional pound of salt over 7 days as you change your diets as not to shock your system.

Nutrients: 2,000 mg. Vitamin C (3 times a day)

100 mg. Vitamin B-complex, (3 times a day)

2 tablespoons spirulina or Heal Thyself Nutritional Formula (3 times a day)

wheatgrass (4 ounces daily with 1 quart of water)

2 cloves of garlic with the juice of lemon and 8-16 ounces of distilled water

Come off of all flesh immediately.

Drink 1 tablet of Rejuvenation Clay to 16 ounces of distilled water.

Diet: Maintain 75% Live and 25% steamed food diet or 100% Live (uncooked)

Anti-Cancer Formula

Herbs: Red clover, chaparrell, echinacea

Juices: Beets, green vegetables, kale, spinach, 12-16 ounces Green Vegetable juice daily

Baths: Warm water bath for 20 minutes, then take a shower alternating temperatures from warm to cool.

Other: Apply clay pack over cancerous area at least 3-7 times a week. During the last 4-9 days of your fast, take Sonne #7 and #9 (Bentonite clay ash). This will provide deeper cleansing of the colon by drawing out longtime toxins. Follow directions on Sonne package. Supplement with two enemas a day.

Nutrients: Follow the Nutrients and Dietary recommendations for Acquired Immune Deficiency Syndrome.

Avoid Flesh and Dairy.

Arthritis — Bone Builder

Herbs: Oatstraw, alfalfa, dandelion

Juices: Turnip (for bones), green vegetables

Baths: Warm water bath; soak 30 minutes; total massage. Add 1 to 2 pounds of Epsom salt to bath.

Other: Apply clay over aches and pains. Massage peanut oil on painful areas.

Drink 1 tablespoon of clay to 12 to 16 ounces of distilled water 3 to 7 times a week.

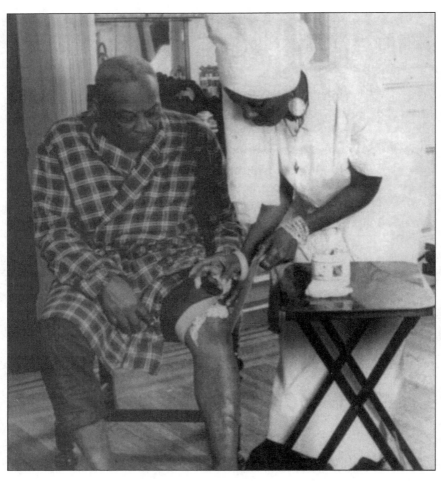

Diabetes

Herbs: Blueberry leaves, goldenseal, yarrow, marshmallow

Juices: String beans and all other green vegetable juices (2 cups); cucumber juice (2 cups); 1-2 artichokes; 2 bunches watercress; 2 bunches parsley

Baths: Salt bath using 2-4 pounds of Epsom salt; stay in tub.

Other: For 20-30 minutes, place a clay application over pancreas; 50% of diet should consist of freshly pressed juices; 50-100% of diet should be raw (uncooked) foods; avoid eating, as in all other cases, when the sun goes down, in order not to overwork the body.

Avoid Flesh, Fried, Dairy, and Sugar and White Flour products.

High Blood Pressure

Herbs: Vervain, goldenseal (Should be taken for only 14 days and then off for 14 days, so as not to deplete the B vitamins from the body.)

Juices: Leeks, garlic

Baths: Warm water bath *without salt*. Soak 15 minutes.

Other: 2-3 enemas weekly or colon deblocker 3 times a week Herbal laxatives and enemas will aid digestion.

Avoid Flesh, Fried and Fast Foods. Avoid cayenne, ginger, celery and salt baths until blood pressure is stable.

Indigestion

Herbs: Peppermint

Juices: 2 cups cabbage to 4 to 8 ounces of Green Juice.

Baths: Warm water baths; soak 20 minutes; massage abdomen.

Other: Drink 3 glasses of lemon water before bath; for exercise, try leg raises (15-25), sit-ups and deep breathing.

Men's Formula

Herbs: Saw palmetto berries, burdock

Juices: Cherry, cranberry

Baths: 30-45 minutes in 4 pounds salt bath; steam baths for 1 hour to 30 minutes.

Other: Clay packs over reproductive organs, cover with gauze overnight.

Nerve Blockage

Herbs: Hops, chamomile, mint

Juices: Celery, cucumber

Baths: 2-4 pounds Epsom salt in a hot bath every other day for 30 minutes; sleep right after bath.

Avoid brown and white sugar.

Nervous Breakdown

Herbs: Valerian (boil 15 minutes), wood betony (steep for 2 hours), gota kola (feeds the brain)

Juices: Celery, cucumber

Baths: 2-4 pounds Epsom salt in a hot bath every other day for 30 minutes; sleep right after bath.

Other: To substitute food alternatives to prevent re-occurrence of the above dis-eases.

Overweight

Herbs: Chickweed, fennel

Juices: Cucumber, parsley

Baths: 2 pounds Dead Sea salt or 4 pounds Epsom salt,

1 cup ginger (Use freshly pressed, but only if you do not have high blood pressure.)

Other: Lecithin (3 times a day), Heal Thyself Formulas 1, II, and III; 30 minutes of daily exercise; fire breaths 100 times (4 rounds)

Avoid eating foods once the sun sets, unless you are eating fruits and vegetables.

Respiratory Problems (Asthma/Hay fever/Colds/Allergies/ Shortness of Breath/Fevers.)

Herbs:	Eucalyptus, mullein
Juices:	Scallions, red radishes, pineapples, grapefruit, lemons, oranges
Baths:	Add peppermint, eucalyptus or camphor to bath; rub on chest and back; put a few drops of oil on tongue (with 25 deep breaths).
Other:	50-100 deep breaths (2-3 times a day)
Note:	A fever is just an extreme cold that has not been handled and decongested properly.
Fevers:	Take enema for 3 days with 3 to 4 tablespoons organic apple cider vinegar. Taking herbal laxative for 3 days of cascara 1-2 tablets, has been useful for children; 3 tablets for adults.

Avoid Flesh and Dairy; eat minimal starches.

The Bob Law Mucus Buster

To eliminate chronic, mucus congestion

- Blend together: 3 tablespoons of organic apple cider vinegar, juice of one freshly pressed grapefruit, juice of one lemon, and 2 drops of pure peppermint oil.
- Drink 4 ounces of warm water after consumption. After drinking, do 50-100 fire breaths (rapid breathing). Take for 7-14 days.

Skin Eruptions

Herbs:	1 teaspoon goldenseal for a cycle of 14 days on and 14 days off
Juices:	Beets, green vegetables, kale, spinach, etc.
Baths:	Alfalfa or goldenseal bath using 1 quart of tea.
Other:	Clay bath over entire body, dry and wash; apply aloe gel to skin.

Avoid Fried foods and Flesh.

Women's Formula

Herbs: Red clover, goldenrod, comfrey, motherwort

Juices: Cherry, cranberry

Baths: 30-45 minutes in 4 pounds Epsom salt bath; steam bathe for 15-30 minutes.

Other: Clay packs over reproductive organs; cover with gauze overnight.

Avoid Fried foods and Flesh.

With each natural suggestion, Purge! Take 1-2 enemas each week and/or an herbal laxative.

Detox on 1 to 4 ounces of fresh wheatgrass 3-7 times a week. With all your Natures Cures, it is suggested that you take 2-3 enemas or herbal laxatives weekly until dis-ease has been arrested.

Nature Cures for Our Children

As a mother and responsible, wholistic parent of 3 children, I acted as my children's personal on-the-job healer throughout their lives. I worked diligently to prevent them from having childhood dis-eases such as colds, ear infections, pneumonia, respiratory ailments, constipation, colic, mumps, measles and chicken pox, and equally worked with nature to increase their memory, concentration, serenity, intelligence and basic good nature. I prepared green vegetable juice with spirulina and wheatgrass. They ate vegetables protein and drank vegetable calcium forms as illustrated in this text. I built up their immune system with garlic, lemons, aloes and bitters. I also gave them salt baths, massages, performed mini-prayer services and limited television viewing. I surrounded them with loving and caring people so they might grow into wholistic, Health-conscious adults and so pass Natural Laws to the next generation, thereby, growing people who are dis-ease free from their very roots.

Children must avoid sugar and junk food. They must also drink a pint to a quart of water daily to cleanse internally.

When I was not as watchful due to life's many ills and distractions, and my children fell short and acquired dis-ease, I aided them to wellness by wrapping them up in nature ways. My children are now adults. My youngest, Ali, is 20, my middle child Sherease Maat, is 22 and my eldest, Supa Nova, is 25. We survived by the help of nature's cures. If your children are challenged and you have the courage to support them with nature's help, then adhere to the following, wellness formulas. You may work with your child's pediatrician as you embrace nature's way; it's your choice.

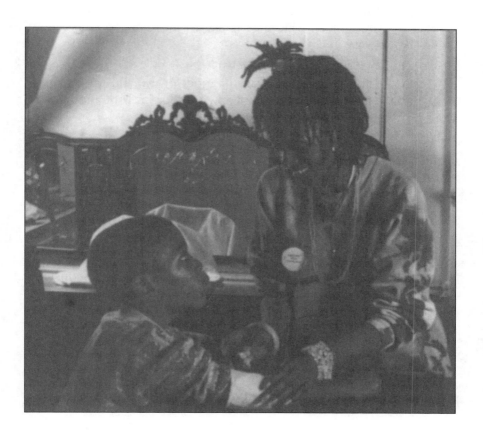

Colds and Fevers

Herbs: Peppermint, fennel, and ¼ teaspoon powdered goldenseal for 7 days (1 teaspoon to 1 cup of warm water).

Juice: 1 grapefruit and 2 oranges together. Add 3-6 drops of liquid Kyolic or juice ¼-1 teaspoon of horseradish and have your child drink it down followed by drinking 4-8 ounces of room temperature distilled water.

Baths: 1 pound Epsom or Dead Sea salt bath; add eucalyptus and peppermint oil to child's chest, back, and a few drops to bath.

Colon: Whenever one has a fever or cold, constipation is present.
Cleansing: For the next 2-3 days, serve your child a bowl of okra or give the little one an enema or herbal laxative to purge out all the backed up accumulated wastes.

Nutrients: Take *Heal Thyself Formula I*. Add 1-2 teaspoons to fresh vegetable or fruit juice. (Take 2 times a day to keep energy up).

Food: 50% vegetable and 50% fruit for 2-3 days.

The above formula also is good for eye and ear infection (Apply clay above and below eyes, or in front and back of ear lobe if congested.)

Clay: Mix 1 tablespoon of clay to 1 tablespoon of pressed ginger and make into a gauze and place on chest. Place tape on both sides to keep in place. Let dry for 2-4 hours or overnight, then shower off. For sprains, bruises or skin eruptions, apply clay with gauze and shower daily until your child has returned to wellness.

Flower Essences: Take Bach flower remedies or other flower essences for emotional imbalances.

Avoid animal calcium such as cow's milk, ice-cream or eggs. Consume only calcium made from vegetable juices, almond, sesame or soya milk.

Constipation

Check your child a few times a week. S/he should eliminate 2-4 times daily.

Herbs: Senna, peppermint

Juices:	Freshly pressed pear, apple, grapefruit and prune
Baths:	Warm water bath
Other:	Okra, vegetable salads, sprouts; rebounder daily 10 minutes
Exercise:	Use rebounder (trampoline) daily; jump for joy 10 minutes a day to unblock.

Avoid starch for 7 days; then eat whole grains in moderation.

| *Water*: | Drink 1 pint of warm distilled water daily. |

Hyperactivity Learning Disabilities

Herbs:	Chamomile, gota kola
Nutrients:	25 mg. Vitamin B-Complex
	1 teaspoon spirulina (brain food) 2 to 3 times a day with fresh fruit or vegetable juice
Juices:	1 celery stalk, 2 cucumber, 3-4 carrots.
Baths:	Add 4 teaspoons of chamomile and hops to 1 quart water. Steep 4 hours; and add to tub. Use 2 pounds bath salt in warm water.
Other:	15 mg. Vitamin B, 3 times a day; Formula I (or 1 teaspoon spirulina) and Formula III, 3 times a day; eliminate all sugar, natural and unnatural, from diet.

Avoid brown or white sugar. For sweets, consume only natural sugars in the form of fresh fruits.

Beauty Foods to be taken Internally and Externally

Here are foods that can be taken internally and externally for health and beauty. Healing can be fun.

Apply sliced cucumbers over eyelids to prevent puffy and bloodshot eyes. To reduce swelling, cover eyes and rest for 15 minutes.

Lemons, limes or grapefruit; drink juice of lemon or lime with 2 grapefruits followed by 8 ounces of distilled water.

Avocado Facial

Full body scrub:

• 1 cup each of water & oats with 2 cups cornmeal.

Mix together and put in bath. Scrub with loofah or scrub over full body and shower.

- Scrub rough blemished areas of elbows, knees, face and feet. Do not use on sensitive skin.

Benefits:

- Cleanses & nourishes skin

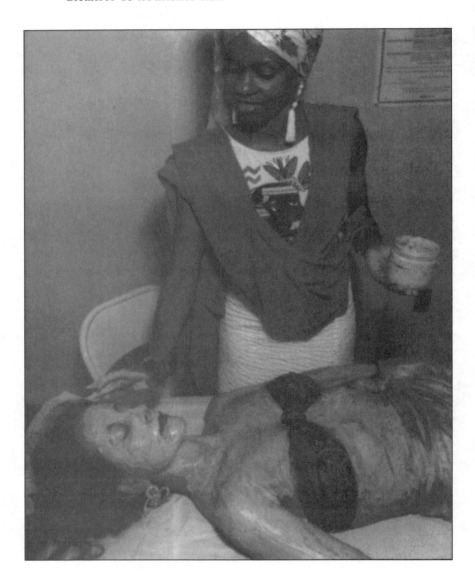

Fourteen

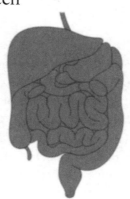

Colon
Therapy

COLON THERAPY — also called colon hygiene, a colonic or colon lever-age — is a thorough form of hydrotherapy (water cure) for the large intestines. It has the ability to restore the entire body system by gently washing the colon clean. Colonic therapy should be administered by a trained, colonic therapist. This is someone who knows the proper amounts and temperatures of water to use and appropriate herbal mixtures and solutions to add to the water for respiration of friendly bacteria in the colon and rejuvenation of tissues.

A colonic therapist also knows other essentials of the procedure, such as administering reflexology on the feet, massaging the abdomen and recommending the proper breathing patterns to the person receiving the colonic.

Basically, 10-15 gallons of purified water is used. As when taking an enema, a tube is inserted into the anus. By using more water suspended at a greater height than an enema, the colonic irrigation becomes a deeper and more thorough cleansing. The water flows into the anus, up into the descending colon area, across the transverse colon area, down into the ascending colon area and finally to the cecum. The cecum (the end of the large intestines) is where large amounts of unfriendly bacteria hibernate and can cause harm to the entire body system. There are nerve endings in the colon (large intestines) that correspond to every organ in the body. Therefore, washing the colon provides cleansing and rejuvenation for the other organs as well.

The Colon

During one colonic session, one to five pounds of old, impacted waste is eliminated. By cleansing the colon, you purge 90% of disease-causing bacteria out of the body. A colonic also cleanses tissues that have been penetrated by poisons. It improves lymphatic circulation.

I especially recommend taking a colonic or a series of colonics during the time of seasonal changes to keep the body functioning at top performance. Depending on your needs and state of health, the use of colonic therapy, along with my other recommendations for purification and natural living, should put you on your path to 'Healing Thyself.'

There are connective points in the colon, which correspond with the various inner organs of the body. As you cleanse the colon with the use of colonic irrigation (hydrotherapy), you begin to heal those various diseased areas of the body. Colonic irrigation along with nutritional guidance and healing exercise can eliminate diseases such as: high blood pressure, edema, skin eruptions, asthma, headaches, hay fever, Fe/male genital disorders, and depression.

Tumors and cysts located in the female reproductive organs and breast are in epidemic proportion. In chronic cases, the end result of this health imbalance is a hysterectomy (a complete removal of the uterus) and mastectomy (removal of the breast). With a holistic program of colon cleansing and nutritional guidance, this problem can be eradicated.

Normal bowel movements should be twice a day if you have two (2) small or large meals daily or three (3) eliminations if taking three (3) meals. The body goes through digestive assimilation and elimination with each meal. If this process, for any reason, does not occur, then you have constipation, which means disease is manifesting or has manifested within your physical, emotional and spiritual body. Take plenty of okra, if constipated, as well as olive oil with lemon water to alleviate the problem or take a bowl of okra, 2-3 times a week, if constipated as well as 1-2 tablespoons of Castor oil, 1-2 tablespoons of cold-pressed Olive oil with the juice of lemon with 8-12 ounces of distilled water.

Did you know? Jesus (Yeshua) used the gourd and the reed upon a branch of a tree to cleanse his inner parts (colon). Cleanliness is next to Godliness.

Bowel Elimination

The Squatting Posture

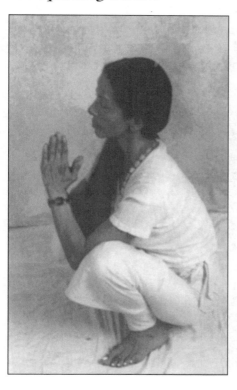

The squatting posture is a natural part of the cultures of Afrika, India and China. The squat is applied during times of rest, washing clothes, preparing meals and, most of all, for the elimination of waste. In cultures where the squat is used frequently, people generally do not suffer from genital disorders. In western countries such as Europe and America, use of the squat as a relaxant and/or healer is virtually unknown. The result is that people there are suffering a great deal with many of the diseases listed earlier.

As per experience, Queen Afua recommends the use of the squatting stool™ during elimination. This stool aids the body by elevating the feet when placed in front of the toilet.

The commercial toilets now in use are a hindrance to the natural functions, for the legs are hanging in line or slightly lower than the hips, causing blockage and making the body work harder through straining, resulting in constipation and hemorrhoids.

Use of the squatting technique, as well as the squatting stool™, is of great importance to aid elimination in the hydrotherapy (bath) room. Better elimination is beneficial toward relief from the above-mentioned ailments.

The Artful Way of Elimination

Step 1:   While sitting on toilet, squat with one or both legs.

Step 2:   Inhale breath for four (4) counts; exhale for eight (8) counts.

Step 3:   On your elimination while inhaling, fill your being with all the goodness there is.

Step 4:   On the exhale, let go and let God, as you release deeply all the negativity in your body, mind, and spirit.

Then sit very still for a moment and feel the peace of your release.

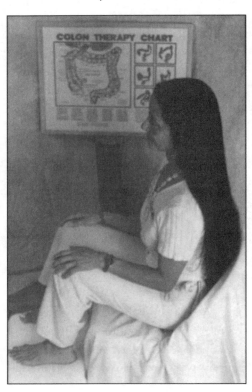

Fifteen

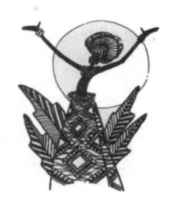

In Celebration of Women: Full Women Free

ALL WE WANT to do here is to be Full Women Free.
We can't be Full and Free, if we drip, drop, drip, drop uhh,
We just want to be as free and full as the Roaring Ocean
The Blazin' Sun & Full Moon and Wide Earth and High
Mountains and Space.

We just want to be Natural Women.
Those women who created the pyramids,
that still stand to the heavens.
Those women who lived off the herbs & bushes
& berries & You, Creator!

Those women who did not bleed.
Not the first women.
We want to be free to dance the dances of joy and sing songs of
bliss and say words of power and touch lives so deep, so sweet.

We don't want no more pain,
We don't want to give no more pain.
No more bleeding, cryin', weepin', moaning.
I can't use no PMS, no more tumors resting in my nest!

I'm gonna Free Me from my bondage and who said I gotta be
cursed anyway?

Oh, it's that cycle again.
Oh goodness, oh gracious.
There's a war going on in me!
Uhh, I've been wounded 1, 3, 5, 6, 7 days!

Oh no don't take my womb!
Give me back my womb! My nest!
I gotta swirl with my nest. A growth!

Leave my breast alone.
Let me be, let me be.
I gotta dance with my breast.
All I want to do here and now is to be
Full Women Free.

Natural Women, Women Sacred, Women Divine,
Women Loving, Women Gracious, Potent and Kind,
Women Clean, Women Whole, WOMEN HEALED!

Whatever you want to be as a Woman, go on and be.
Can't nobody put no limits on me!
If you want to be an Artist, go on and be.
If you want to be a Scientist, go on and be.
If you want to be a Mother Writer, go on and be.
If you want to make soup, or own a business or
do cartwheels down the street, go on and be.

Being you're so powerful, so purified, so spiritual.
You can be anything you want to be!
If you want to be President of a country, child,
go on and be.

Whatever I wanna do and be ...
Mother, Father God already gave it to me.

We, women, just want to be and we're going to be and
We are Full Women Free.

Cause if I don't feel full within myself,
l just might lose myself;
and I love you Free Women.

I don't want to lose any of you.
I don't want to lose any part of me.
I love all of Me!
Free Women, go on and be!

F R E E

Be Healed.

This poem is dedicated to Heal Thyself Women's Research Group for
Living a Pure Life, for their efforts of constantly purifying for a period
of one to seven months on fruits, vegetables, live juices, and monthly
fasting, prayer and constant purification of the soul, thoughts and heart.

For believing, knowing and living the truth that women need not
bleed and suffer monthly and have the power to bring their menses
from 6 days to 4, from 4 days to 1.

Thank you for being a living witness and enduring until the end:

Kamari Aduke	Pearl L. Boissiere
Merlene Byron	Arlene Crosby
Jacquelyn Crossland	Khadijah Dunn
Shirley Edwards	Etherine Fortune
Lynda Johnson Garrett	Colleen Goldberg
Deanna Hope	Tracy Jerigen
Isa Karriem	Marcia Lilly
Akua Morris	lbon M. Muhammad
Omani Peterson	Khadijah Rahman
Joy Jon San (Illustrator)	Fikriyyah Sharrief
Mimi Strum	Shaunderion White
Adamen (Lenora Peterson)	

And for Elder Micah for inspiring this sacred cleansing program so that other women would no longer have to suffer.

Special thanks to the Mothers of Purification: Queen Esther, Lady Prema, Dr. Abena Asantawaa, Mother Lucille Shepherd, and Fatimahta Adegoke.

Choices

These words will be found in the screenplay, *In All My Born Days* by Ayoka Chenzra. A mystic healer, played by Queen Afua, speaks these divine words to a young female child just coming into her 'woman-ness' and lets her know she has choices to be well and whole or ill, imbalanced and in pain.

"You are a woman. This is a most sacred time for you; a time of renewal, a time for power. Women of old did not suffer. They would go to themselves, and pray, heal, receive spiritual messages for guidance and give thanks for their womaness."

"The modern woman with her impure life style suffers during her moon 4, 5, 6, 7, and sometimes 8 days."

"During your monthly moon, a message from the pituitary goes down to the ovaries and tells them to release an egg, which travels down the fallopian tubes. If your body is free from toxins, then you release a white milky fluid, but if your body is full of poisons from devitalized processed foods and bad thoughts, then you may suffer for days and days."

"Rainbow," the mystic said to the young woman, "you must lead a clean, healthy life, or else when you reach my age, you will suffer with tumors, cysts and early aging."

"I love you, Rainbow. Take care."

Queen Afua

WHERE ARE YOU?

Are You A Full Woman Free?

Over the years, I've found a direct relationship between dietary habits and the health of female organs.

Note: As we travel down the recommendations, it indicates a breakdown of women's health and a decline of healthy living.

Ideal Health

No female problems (vaginal disorders)

Menses for 1-3 days

Inner peace and harmony

- Whole foods, fasting, enemas, herbs
- Daily exercise
- No flesh or fried foods
- Limited starches
- Bowel movements 3 or more times a day; stools long, light-colored, full and easy to eliminate

Decline of Health

Beginning Stages of Degeneration

Prolapsed colon causes prolapsed uterus, which induces lower back pain, which results in 3-5 day menses, which causes vaginal itch/discharge.

- Flesh foods (fish, chicken), nighttime eating, lack of exercise
- Dairy and starches
- Two or fewer bowel movements

2ⁿᵈ Stage of Degeneration

Cysts and fibroid tumors

Caesarean section in birthing (difficult birthing)

Lack of sexual orgasm (due to blockage/poor circulation)

Menses of 5-8 days or acute menses of 8 days to 2 weeks

- Flesh foods (beef, pork)
- Drugs (orthodox and unorthodox)
- Continued neglect of exercise
- Dairy, starch, sugar
- One bowel movement: short, hard stool
- Kidney stones

3rd Stage of Degeneration

Tumors (hysterectomy)

Removal of the uterus; sterility

Lack of sexual enjoyment or stimulation

Suppressed emotions; discomfort with femaleness

- Continued negligence of emotional, physical condition
- One bowel movement a day or a few times a week: hard, short, grassy

Vaginal Regeneration

Women: stop feeding your tumors. Save your uterus and save your breasts.

Foods that create and feed tumors or cysts are flesh products, such as all meats (pork, beef, chicken and fish), dairy products such as milk, cheese and ice cream. Avoid fried foods and starches.

A diet heavy in these foods creates 4-8 days or up to 2 weeks of bleeding. Usually, when a woman receives surgery to remove a tumor or cyst, it grows back in 1-2 years because she, in her ignorance, continues to eat the above-mentioned foods.

Once, she eliminates the above foods, the tumor either will be eliminated or will not develop again. If a woman has a tumor or cyst and she discontinues eating foods that help a tumor or cyst to strive, the tumor or cyst begins to die out and comes out of the woman through the vagina in small or large lumps of what appears to be mucus.

The regeneration and purification process is speeded up if she takes large amounts of vegetable juices, spirulina, wheatgrass and a women's herbal formulas of goldenrod, red clover, red raspberries, and dong quai (a Chinese herb that strengthens the uterus, builds blood and is high in Vitamin B_{12}).

Add 3 teaspoons of each herb to 3-5 cups of water. Steep overnight. Strain and drink in the morning.

For further information and study, read Womb Wisdom in *Sacred Woman: A Guide for Healing the Feminine Body, Mind and Spirit* by Queen Afua.

Basic Regeneration Diet consists of:
- Live fruits and vegetables, vegetable broth and vegetable soups.
- Please, no starch, even if whole grains, until problem is totally eliminated.

Bless Your Dis-ease Away

Emotionally, you must consistently release anger, frustration and disappointment out of your vagina and mind. Release thoughts of anyone who you feel has hurt you and take the experience as a lesson. Forgive that person in order for you to release the person or experience out of your womb along with the tumor.

A good time or way to release emotionally and revitalize yourself spiritually is during your healing bath. While in bath, massage, breathe, nurture and bless your pain and disease away. Fill your womb with peace and mentally bathe your womb with green light for healing and pink light for love. Each month, thereafter, you will bleed one day less. The more you love your vagina and your womaness, the sweeter and more harmonious the children who can come through your sacred canal will be. The planet's salvation depends on you loving yourself. It may take you months or years to bring your bleeding from five days to one day, a half day to one hour. But, don't give up, for healing is close at hand.

Chant daily and pray for women who have buried their wombs. Women, Heal Ourselves! Save Our Uterus! Save Our Wombs! Save Our Uterus! Save Our Wombs! Save Our Uterus!

In order to receive the Creator's blessing in the heights, we, women, must be willing to live without flesh and the by-products of the beast. When an animal sheds its blood for our desires, we, too, shall shed our blood, in this case, monthly for the women. As Kahlil Gibran states in his book, *The Prophet*, "When you kill a beast, say to him in your heart, 'by the same power that slays you, I, too, am slain: and I, too, shall be consumed. For the law that delivered you into my hand, shall deliver me into a mightier hand.' "

Toxic-filled Women (Heavy Bleeding)	*Purified Women* (Light Bleeding)
3-8 days or more clotting	1-60 minutes to 1-2 days; no clotting
Depression	Gaiety
Mood swings	Mental peace, harmony
Loss of vital life fluids	Retention of vital fluids
Low energy	High energy
Agitated	Strong concentration
Infertility	Increased fertility
Poisoned vagina-clotting, odor	Pure odor-free vagina
Quick to anger, violent temper	Healthy, happy and beautiful disposition
White vaginal discharge	Clear vaginal discharge

Depending on the length of your menses, it will determine the intensity of either expression.

If you find that you have cleansed yourself with nature's tools for weeks and months and your tumor is still strong within, and if you choose surgery, your healing after surgery will be expedient. If you live naturally, thereafter, your tumor, in most cases, will not return. Continue in this way for 1-2 years and you will no longer be feeding the tumors and cysts.

Loosen your thoughts, your hips and Temple gate. As we enter into our healing and change our diets, we also should apply this simple message. We must stop constricting ourselves. Take off those tight pants and girdles for improved circulation of oxygen, blood flow and nutritional acceptance. When in the privacy of your home, spread your thighs and allow Shu, the angel of air, to wash your sacred chamber, as you breathe deeply 50 or more fire breaths. During this time, send messages of beauty and love to and through your divine canal. When able, let RA, the angel of fire (sun), recharge and bathe you with its rays of light and healing. Go outside daily, and get a sunbath 30 minutes to an hour. If you have a private yard or you are at a beach with women to guard you, you may spread your thighs open to the direction of the sun. Closing your eyes, visualize the sun rays recharging you internally. Be at peace with your womaness and observe your healing taking place.

No more hysterectomies. No more drugs. No more surgery. No more pain. I address the area of supreme healing to women as in time of old when we were healthy, happy and whole.

Know that by nature you are a beautiful flower, a healing herb a lotus-like mind, body and spirit. From birth, you come with sacred earth medicine to heal yourself.

For a more comprehensive study on womb wellness, read Chapter 24 in *Sacred Woman: A Guide To Healing the Feminine Body, Mind and Spirit.*

A Special Message to Breast-Feeding Mothers

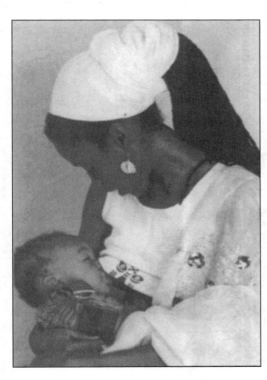

You should strive to breast-feed for 1-3 years (if not for the full time, at least part time). Mothers should follow a natural mucus-less diet so that the baby is free of colic, constipation, constant crying and cradle cap. Mothers should eat fresh fruits, vegetables (especially okra), vegetable juice of 4-5 carrots, 2 cucumbers, 2 turnips, or juice of dark green vegetables i.e. kale ½ cup, broccoli ½ cup, spinach ¼ cup and turnip ½ cup, and vegetarian proteins such as peas, beans, sprouts, tofu, seeds and nuts. If you are a meat-eater, eat only baked non-shell fish.

Take advantage of the following nutrients: TwinLab

Yeast Liquid (2 tablespoons), spirulina (2 teaspoons to 2 tablespoons) and 500-1,000 mg. of Vitamin C, all to be taken 2-3 times a day with fresh vegetables or fruit juice. Drink 1 quart of distilled water daily to keep your milk and your spirit flowing like water. Also utilize vegetarian calcium sources in the form of soya milk, nut and sesame seed milk, carrot and turnip juice, and oatstraw, dandelion, alfalfa, and comfrey herbal teas.

Mothers: Take steam baths to keep the pores cleansed and the nerves relaxed. If mother is upset, she will poison the baby. So, husband, nurture and love the mother of your child, the love of your life.

Here are some other things brothers can do:

- Prepare woman's bath once a week and place her into the tub. Remember: To serve is to be served.
- Bring her flowers.
- Massage her gently with 3 parts olive oil, 1 part Vitamin E.

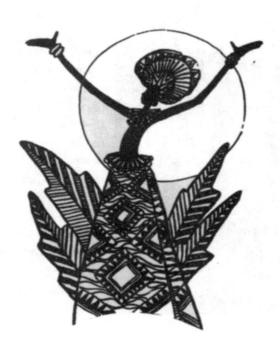

The 12 Principles of Divine Sacred Woman

These 12 Principles are for Women who strive to be Healed and Whole. The woman is the center of the home. If she takes her sacredness as a woman seriously, the children and husband (mate) will also be functioning in Divine Order.

   As you affirm these principles daily for yourself, you will steadily experience yourself opening up like a beautiful lotus.

AS A SACRED WOMAN: I am the highest physical and spiritual projection of *woman-consciousness*. I represent the abundance of life in health, wealth, love and beauty.

AS A SACRED WOMAN: I embody grace, dignity and majesty—at all times.

AS A SACRED WOMAN: I epitomize the highest aspects of the feminine principle in my great love of being a *Woman*.

AS A SACRED WOMAN: I nurture myself through the nurturing of others.

AS A SACRED WOMAN: I manifest the highest principles of *spirit, mind*, and *body*, through my transformation of *thought, word* and *deed*.

AS A SACRED WOMAN: I can never be abused by *man, woman* or *child* for I represent the active presence and power of the Almighty Creator.

AS A SACRED WOMAN: I have the power to *heal* with a *glance*, a *smile* or a *word*.

AS A SACRED WOMAN: I am the ORIGINAL HEALER, who calls upon the Creator's creation, (the Elements AIR, FIRE, WATER AND EARTH) to heal *physically, mentally and spiritually*, for I am the Great-Granddaughter of MOTHER NATURE herself!

AS A SACRED WOMAN: I beam and radiate my *inner* Divinity, by adoring my *outer* Being with garments befitting my Royal form. I would never dress in the clothing of my masculine counterpart, for then I *surrender my power! my tools!*

AS A SACRED WOMAN: I don't kill living creatures for food. I am a vegetarian-fruitarian by nature; my food contains the breath of life. I take into my body Temple live fruits, vegetables, nuts, seeds, juices and herbs for "life comes only from life; life gives only unto itself."

AS A SACRED WOMAN: I endeavor to transform my domestic atmosphere into a PARADISE!!! My environment radiates my inner tranquility.

The very walls of my home (temple) reflect the divine sanctity and safety of the womb. So, whoever enters into my temple shall be lifted to their heights.

AS A SACRED WOMAN: I am ever striving to resurrect and exalt the divinity of my mate and counterpart. I recognize that my inner balance must manifest externally in my relationship with MAN, if the true potential of the Higher Self is to be made known to me.

Upon each rising and setting of the sun, woman or man must unite with self, become whole through Natural Living Principles. We marry ourselves, become one with our self in Body, Mind and Spirit in order to reflect that external reflection. I affirm these 12 Principles so that I may be living more each day, the heights and the perfection of the Divine Sacred Woman.

I, _____, accept my divine position and responsibility as a Divine Sacred Woman on _____.

"Shine, You Brilliant Woman, First Mother, Healer, Lover of the Universe."

Sixteen

Hydrotherapy: Water Baptism

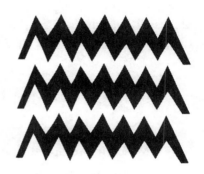

Xu-kua, ab-kua... I am glorious, I am pure...
Ancient Khametian prayer

THE WATER ELEMENT was very sacred during the First Civilization of the Nile Valley. The Khamites used a great deal of water for Spiritual Baptisms to wash away the ills, to bring forth life and to prepare one to enter the Mystery Systems, which were part of the entrance course into knowledge of the Most High. To support this, it is said in *Ancient Egypt Light of the World* by Gerald Massey, that we might call the Khamites very particular Baptists. In the first 10 gates into the great dwelling of Ausar — the Resurrection Principle — the initiate is purified at least 10 times over, in 10 separate baptisms, in 10 different waters, corresponding to the different states of man's spirit, in waters blessed by the Neteru, in which the Neteru had been washed to make the water holy. The initiate would say, "May I be protected by seventy purifications." In the rituals, it is said, "I purify myself at the great stream of the galaxy. That which is wrong in me is pardoned and the spots upon my body, upon the earth are washed away. I come, that I may purify this soul of mine in The Most High Degree."

Water is as sacred now, in the Motherland of Afrika as in our hearts, as it was then. When you enter into someone's home, to this day oftentimes, the first thing you are given is water. Water represents life (Ankh). The oldest word for Life in Afrikan language is NK, usually spelled *Ankh*. Nk is rendered a wave of water and a sieve. This establishes water as a primary element of the Life Force. The sieve catches all impurities.

As researched by SEN-UR HRU ANKH RA SEMAHJ SE PTAH

HETEP PTAH TEMPLE

Healing Water Prayer

Oh Father, Mother God, these waters that I bathe and wash Myself in are Spiritual and Holy, for they are your Waters.

Baptize me in your Holy Divine Waters.

Direct my course, as I cleanse with this Purifying Tool. Purify Me, Oh Creator of the Universe.

Cleanse me from within and without.

Help me to let go of all that is not you;

All that is not truth.

Allow this Holy Water to scrub all my sickness, pain and confusion away.

I now wash my head and there is light.

I wash my heart and there is love.

I wash my body Temple, so that I may be drawn closer and closer to you.

Hold me in your arms, Great and Divine Father, Mother.

Baptize me with your Love.

Heal me with your Love.

Engulf me with your water.

Queen Afua

Apply this prayer with the fire (sun) bath, earth (clay or sand) bath, air bath and water (ocean) bath.

This Water Prayer is dedicated to Baba Ishangi for teaching me the ancient Afrikan Power of Spiritual Bathing. Pray before and during your water healing (baths, enemas, colonics, nose rinses and showers). In place of Father, Mother God, put in the term you use for The Most High.

A Few More Words About Water...

I recommend that you read *Colon Health Key To Vibrant Life* by Norman W. Walker. Mr. Walker, like me, was a colon therapy student of Dr. Robert A. Wood, a healer who lived to the age of 88 and was going strong to the end. My study under Dr. Wood, as well as my personal health experience, has led me to understand and be very grateful for the element water, for water therapy has restored and saved my life.

Baths

Soaking in a warm tub will enable the body to release toxins through the skin. Epsom salt or Dead Sea salt is recommended (unless you have

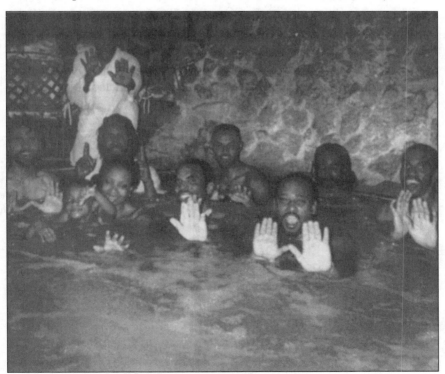

high blood pressure). Use 2-4 pounds of salt and soak in tub for 30 minutes. A few drops of eucalyptus oil is recommended for general use and, especially, when there is congestion in the lungs. If you have a cold or mucus congestion, massage peppermint or camphor oil into your chest while bathing. Be sure to keep hands away from face as not to burn eyes as massaging oil into the chest, etc. Also, add a few drops into the bath water. See the following chart and refer to Chapter 3 for suggested oils in bath.

Scrub body with loofah brush and wash with natural soap or Queen Afua's Rejuvenating Clay to open and cleanse pores and allow the body to breathe. You can massage your feet and body during your bath, always working upward toward the heart.

Take a warm bath or choose to take a brisk, cool shower daily. Take a warm shower if you have a cold or respiratory problems. Dry body well and anoint with oil.

To set the stage for profound self-healing, do the following: Take deep breaths or burn oil in a heating dish. Place a small candle to light the way in the hydrotherapy (bath) room. Also place fresh flowers to beautify your transcendental experience or, prior to the bath, burn a small amount of frankincense and myrrh or sage brush, for spiritual cleansing, and turn off to limit effects on lungs in enclosed room, and open window for a brief time to air out smoke. Burn frankincense and myrrh or sage brush for spiritual cleansing.

Bath oils to consider:

Almond oil - for prosperity.

Camphor - to strengthen psychic/spiritual powers.

Honeysuckle - to promote quick thinking and aid memory.

Hyssop - to purify the atmosphere and the body; increases finances.

Rose oil - for love matters; to inspire peace and harmony.

Spikenard - wear during rituals to the ancient deities of Egypt (Khamit); also anoint sacred objects, such as altars, tools, etc.

How to take an Enema

It is of utmost importance to take a daily enema while on this cleansing. A quart-size enema bag will be sufficient. Fill the bag with warm water. Be sure to test the water temperature on the inside of your wrist. You may want to add 3 tablespoons of organic apple cider vinegar to combat symptoms of respiratory disorders.

Other enema implant suggestions include:

Wheatgrass Enema: Add 1 ounce to 1 quart of water.

Liquid Chlorophyll: Add 3 tablespoons to 1 quart of water.

Lemon/Lime Enema: Add juice of 1 lemon/lime to 1 quart of water. First remove seeds.

Garlic Enema: Empty 2 capsules of garlic or 6-12 drops of liquid Kyolic into 2 quarts of warm water, then into enema bag and mix well.

- Lubricate the nozzle tip of a 1 or 2 quart enema bag with K-Y Jelly or other water-soluble jelly.

- Lie in the tub on your back or on your left side. Insert nozzle into rectum and take in up to 1 cup of water.

- Massage the lower left side of your abdomen. Work especially hard on any lumps or ridged areas that you might feel — these are deposits of fecal matter.

- After 3-4 minutes of massaging, let in more water. Continue to massage across the abdomen and down the right side. This is where the greatest problems occur, so be especially thorough in massaging this area.

- Do not retain the liquid if you feel the need to eliminate. Move to the toilet and release. Then, repeat the procedure.

- While sitting on toilet to eliminate, massage abdominal area from right to left, breathe deeply while inhaling and exhaling.

Most people will expel brown or gray mucus, black fleck-like matter, parasites, and other surprising matter.

For deeper cleansing of old impacted waste, place a stool in front of the toilet, place both feet flatly on stool or sit directly on the toilet seat in the ancient position of a squat.

We must work on our colon through cleansing, enemas, abdominal exercise, proper breathing and prayer until we have 3 bowel movements daily. Once our colons are cleansed, 90% of all disease will no longer plague our bodies.

My cleansing proverb: *Life is a reflection; if you don't like your life, wash your mirror.*

Nose Rinse

If the nasal and sinus passages are unclear, it hinders the flow of oxygen to the brain. This lack of oxygen also affects the eyes and ears. So, clear your nasal and sinus passages and enjoy clearer vision, greater hearing, and a sharper mind.

To prevent and relieve nasal congestion, do nose rinses frequently.

* Fill a small tea pot or neti pot with 1 to 2 cups of water with a pinch of sea salt, or 1 teaspoon of chlorophyll.
* Tilt your head over the sink so the left side of your face is parallel to the sink. Open your mouth and keep it open.
* Place the nozzle of the neti pot at your right nostril and gently pour the water.

If done correctly, the water will flow through and expel through your left nostril. Repeat this procedure, beginning with the head tilting to the right and pouring water into the left nostril, expelling through the right.

Following the nose rinse, do 25-50 full fire breaths.

Fire Breathing is rapid breathing. The purpose of fire breathing is to increase circulation. It also serves to detoxify the body, i.e. organs and blood.

Deep inhalation in as you breathe in through the nose, down through your lungs, into your abdomen, prior to exhaling out from the abdomen, allowing the air to flow through the lungs then through the nose. This movement should be done in quick and strong motions.

If you feel light-headed, then stop breathing and resort to slow, deep inhalations, breathing out another four to eight times before breathing normally.

Seventeen

Exercises for Body, Mind and Spiritual Conditioning

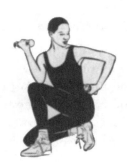

Daily exercise is necessary for a minimum of 15 minutes to a maximum of 1 hour.

FOR THOSE OF you who are experiencing body Temple degeneration such as: numbing out, being tired even after a good night sleep, depressed, but don't know where it's coming from. Maybe you are stuck in a rut. Then, move where you sit; rotate your arms forward and backward, stretch your fingers. Grab some energy, roll the stress out of your neck. Get up and reach for your toes; pick up your life. Swing open the door; step forward and power walk down the street. It's easy—just start where you are, you've got what it takes. Enjoy life, don't hesitate; get moving right now!

Regular exercise, in whatever form you choose, can help you to re-sculpture your life into divine order. Exercise helps you to firm and tone up your mental, physical and spiritual muscles. Exercise enhances longevity as it aids in prevention or elimination of arthritis, aches and pains, etc. It helps to squeeze out bottled up emotions that cause you a sense of serenity.

Exercising gives you the ability to digest food, enjoy life and celebrate people. Observe with each movement that is accompanied with the breath; witness as you move. As you exercise, you will sort out why you created your life conditions and what it will take to resolve, heal-up or grow from the experience. Exercise clears a cluttered mind as it releases mental depression, leaving you with a more positive, productive attitude towards life. Exercise helps you to strengthen relations, creating harmony with whomever you workout within life.

Basic Head-to-Toe Exercise

Full Body Breath -- deep inhalation on a count of 4. Exhale on a count of 8. On the inhalation, extend the abdomen out along with expansion of the rest of the body. As you exhale, contract the abdomen and release the chest. With each breath, relax the body and the mind deeper and deeper.

- As you do any form of exercise, always apply this deep breath to pump life into the blood, nerves, arteries, muscles, lungs and brain. When moving arms, legs or head upwards, inhale. When you move any part of the body downward, exhale.

- Visualize your pores of your skin opening and closing with each breath. Do this full body breath; breathing from head to toe at least 25 to 100 or more times.

- Fire Breathe — For more energy, and increased circulation for mental power, and physical strength. Inhale and exhale rapidly using the abdomen as a quick release pump. Complete 25-100 breaths.

- Legs in 45º angle against the wall (*natural slant board*) 5-10 minutes. Sit ups and leg raises 10-20 times.

- Arm swings 20-40 times front and back in circles and sides.

- Daily walking — 15 minutes — swing your arms as you walk for upper body circulation.

- Neck rolls — 4 times both sides: Shoulders lifts — 10-20 times.

- Pelvic lifts — lying on your back, bend your knees in to prevent lower back pressure. With each movement up, you inhale; with each movement down, you exhale. Example: As your arm moves up towards the ceiling, you inhale the breath; as your arm goes down towards the floor, you exhale.

The breathing process is the same with each movement in all exercise forms.

Massage For Renewal
from Deanna N. Hope

Massage or laying on of hands is an ancient healing art form. It was performed by Ast (Isis), the great mother and her sister, Nebt-Het, in the temple as a healing ritual to reform and resurrect Asar, the king of Khemit (Egypt).

As you visit the ancient temples, you will witness the first reflexology treatments (foot massages), performed as a form of healing and as a way of relaxing the body Temple.

To prevent accumulation of stress and tension throughout the years, I have received massages personally on a weekly basis to maintain a high standard of health. Since I opened my center Heal Thyself in 1982, I have always kept a masseur/masseuse on staff to service the community. Deanna N. Hope was one of such divine staff members who had a healing touch of gold and a healing spirit like that of Nefer Atum the Lotus, an Afrakan term and principle, for the illuminated one. As a result of her Maat (balanced) nature, I requested her to submit a message to inspire you to tune into massage, thereby, making it a part of your holistic health regime for longevity as well as inner and outer beauty.

According to Deanna Hope, the origins of therapeutic massage are rooted in the common instinctual response to hold or rub a hurt or pain. Massage as an art form is as old as civilization itself. It has been used for thousands of years for relaxation, and restoring and promoting health. In some countries, it is even a medical discipline.

Hope continues saying, you will feel, after a good massage, as if you have had a good night's rest. You may even admit to feeling younger. Massage relieves tension, lowers stress levels, improves mental response, increases cardiovascular and internal organ efficiency, flushes out metabolic toxins, and reduces recovery time from injuries.

We are fortunate beings in that we are directly involved in the goings on of our own bodies. We are the best doctors for our own aches, pains and cures. The more in tune you become with yourself, the easier it is to divert discomforts, detect the cause, and direct the cures. As a society at large, we are not taught to be our own doctors or healers...

"A generation has passed in which the treasure of home-grown cures of our legacy of Afrikan knowledge, instilled in our genes and through our elders, grandparents or great-grandparents is bypassed for the 'quick fix' of the local 'drug' store. The more attention we give to this great reserve of intuitive knowledge the less time and money we will spend on doctor bills.

Further, Deanna says, massage as a healing art form is one of those great treasures. It can be as simple as getting a hug to spending hours, if needed, giving yourself a massage, as part of your at-home healing treatment. The more time spent caring and getting to know every part of your body, mind, and spirit, the less time you'll spend doing things that limit your health, strength, and vitality, and believe me, everything around you will help you to maintain the good practices that you follow and emulate in your life.

Sounds to me like the beginning of a bright and beautiful new world, Deanna adds. "Anyone who knows me well can tell you, I love to get a good massage. The very first professional massage I received was so magnificent I enrolled in a one-year course to obtain my license and certification.

"The best way I can describe the benefits of massage is to tell you the many ways it can help you in overcoming debilitating aches, pains, and stresses. One of the first things to remember when you are getting a massage is the importance of relaxation. Both you and the massage therapist will enjoy the fullness of the benefits of the treatment if you relax your mind, body and spirit.

Massage is a very spiritual as well as a physical and mental healing therapy. Our ancestors of ancient Khamit knew well the benefits of this ancient healing art. They studied the body in all aspects — spirit, mind and body — and understood that the balance of the chakras (energy points) and meridians (highways to connecting nerve cells) were key in the developmental and healing processes of the body. They were cognizant that our self-concept in body, mind and spirit affects our breathing, which affects our life and health.

They also developed many other healing art forms, which were later inherited by other cultures that we know today. For instance, what is called Hatha Yoga today comes from the ancient Khamitic form called Het-Hru Yoka.

Basically, the form is centered around the breath or technique of breathing, which is life. Once our breath is centered, through the MRKHT (pyramid) of the nose and diaphragm, all the other areas of the body are also centered. The spirit, which is our earthly connection to the Divine Creator and Knower of All Things, is continually in communication with our Ba (spirit) and our Ka (soul) to manifest its divinity in our Kaat (body).

From pre-conception to birth to all of the stages of our growth and development, the spirit divinely guides our Kaat to develop to the highest physical, mental and spiritual potentials. Whether it be in art, science, dance, or any form the Creator manifests, our Ka (soul) must be attuned or at one with the Divine Spirit in order to develop to the unlimited potentials of the Creator.

As the IAU Khrishna-Christos stated, "Greater things will ye do than me." Therefore, the art and science of massage and HET-HRU Yoka breath therapy facilitates the manifestation of the Kaat (body) to the Divine Spirit.

As we began life, even before conception and growth through childhood and puberty to adulthood, our bodies changed as our mental development grew with the ideas and information our parents, families, and institutions of learning supplied.

It may be very apparent to you how differently the bodies of people born in different areas of the globe develop, not only because of climate, but also because of diet and spiritual mentality as well. One can sometimes clearly place a Western "civilized" physique from that belonging to one of an Afrikan or other person of closer Afrikan ancestry. We can attribute this most readily to the spiritual development of the person, in relation to the adaptation of the individual to the Divine Spirit.

Given the above, without the proper attention given to healthy nutritional habits such as cleansing, fasting, or drinking water, fruit and vegetable juices, and of divine spiritual development, as opposed to religious barbarism, a person will develop the physika (physical and spiritual bodies) to match whatever stage the above has revealed or manifested.

Poor spiritual development, lack of proper cleansing and fasting or unhealthy nutrition will manifest the same in illness and disease, aches, pains and stress. Therefore, proper intuitive spiritual guidance, cleansing, fasting, and eating, plus massage and exercise, and Het-Hru Yoka (breathing) will facilitate the visualizing abilities, which allow us to transform our spirits and bodies as divinely ordained, so that we can bring Divine light energy into the world, through our vehicles. This process allows us to share supreme power.

It is the Divine will of the Creator that at 20, 30, 40, 50, 60, 70, and even according to current health reports up to at least age 120, we should feel at maximum physical potential and divine strength as we did at 20 years of age or even better. The cells in our bodies regenerate entirely every seven years. We can help our bodies to continue this regeneration process by continuing to exercise our Divine Breath in Het-Hru Yoka.

Here is a list of some of the known benefits of massage:
- Opens blood vessels to improve circulation.
- Increases blood supply and nutrition to muscles.
- Greater ease and range of motion.
- Stimulates lymphatic system to help filter bacteria.
- Assists in maintaining chiropractic adjustments and alignments.
- Aids in stress reduction.
- Increases longevity.

In addition to the benefits, of massage, there is one overall objective to keep in mind at all times — and that is love.

Most definitely, without love for yourself and life, no amount of massage, exercise, fasting, cleansing, or purifying will help—to a good degree. These healing efforts are aided a thousandfold when we do it with love. The Great Spirit most definitely helps those who make any effort to help themselves.

Love yourself and know that you are here because of the Love of the Great Spirit who wanted you to be here to enjoy life to its fullest and breathed the breath of life into your soul to make you a living, vibrant and beautiful being.

There are many techniques for massages. In looking for a masseur or masseuse, one should keep in mind the following objective: the importance of a loving, giving, sharing spirit. It is also very important to remember that you get what you put out. We are all reflections of one another.

Here are some massage techniques that you can look for in a therapist or if you are interested in studying a technique on your own.

Swedish Massage

Swedish massage is the systematic and scientific manipulation of the soft tissues of the body. In 1812, P. Henrik Ling, a Swedish physiologist, developed Swedish massage by applying scientifically established principles of anatomy and physiology to Chinese techniques, and combining them with the movements of Swedish gymnastics. The Swedish massage therapist uses kneading, stroking, friction, tapping, and, sometimes, shaking and vibrating parts of the body in order to stimulate circulation, increase muscle tone and create a balance within the structure and function of the muscular, nervous and circulatory systems. In Swedish massage, the general purpose is to increase circulation, remove toxins, improve flexibility and tone the muscles. The therapist should begin with slow, gliding strokes and, gradually, increase in vigor and movement of the limbs for increased range of motion.

Shiatsu

Shiatsu ("Shi" = finger, "Atsu" = pressure) is an Oriental massage in which particular points of the body are pressed to ease aches, pains, tensions, fatigue and symptoms of disease. Pressure is applied to these vital points with fingers, thumbs and palms to bring relief. (Great therapists, like myself, will even use their elbows, knees, whatever works, to remove the discomfort and relieve the pain. Most of all have fun!)

Shiatsu maintains health, vitality and stamina in the body. It strengthens internal organs and prevents energy from getting blocked. Applying pressure to the meridians and chakras opens up the electrical pathways of the nervous system. As you open these points, you release negative energy, toxins, or emotions (chemical, electro-magnetic energy), which helps us to move with greater ease. The therapist should be sensitive to the patient's emotional and stress-related work or life style and help to remove the blocks mentally and spiritually that create tension as well.

Acupressure

Acupressure is similar to Shiatsu. In Shiatsu, the practitioner manipulates various parts of the body. Acupressure differs from Shiatsu in that it consists mainly of pressure-point therapy. Acupressure requires the recipient's participation with the therapists in coordinating the breath with the manipulations. It is a quiet and contemplative form of massage, having profound results. (Like I said, we're all in this together.)

Foot Reflexology

Foot reflexology is a science based on the principle that there are areas in the feet that correspond to every organ, gland and other parts of the body. With specific hand and finger techniques, the feet are "worked" to break down deposits and cause reactions. These reactions could best be described as relaxation, or a return to equilibrium.

Sports Massage

Sports massage focuses on the psychological and physiological effects of exercise. It is geared toward the professional athlete to improve fitness and performance endurance and in the prevention and treatment of injuries.

In conclusion, Deanna says the holistic practitioner who uses massage therapy may apply a combination of all of these techniques as needed. Check your bookstore and also health food stores for books on massage and healing therapies that are best suited for you. I love you—and me. Here's to many days ahead of happiness, health, prosperity, enjoyment and inner joy.

Love, Peace, Blessings and Smiles.

Hatha Yoga

Each person can use Hatha Yoga postures (asanas) to unify mind, body and spirit, and to create inner harmony and peace. Hatha Yoga emphasizes relaxation. It conserves energy rather than expending it, for Yoga eliminates excitement, which adds toxins to the system.

A few minutes of daily practice in total awareness of body and mind will, ultimately, produce a calming state of inner control, a positive mental attitude, and a more energetic and loving spirit.

Suggestions for Yoga Practice

In Yoga, one should never strain. Relax, never force yourself. You will be astonished how many poses you can accomplish by progressively deeper relaxation.

Practice postures out-of-doors or by an open window. If you cannot bend your body into a particular position, don't concern yourself, for tomorrow is another day. Now is the time to cultivate patience.

Movements should be slow, but deliberate in every case. Sudden, jerky movements should be avoided.

Before you begin, it is better to wash and attend to your body functions.

Start with a minute of silent prayer, open your eyes or let them remain closed and begin asanas.

The postures on the following page are Yoga asanas, which you may use in your private sessions at home.

Stretching the body while using the breath helps to release tension and mental stress, and release toxins out of the body.

Om Shanti (Peace)

Ari-Ankh-Ka

Ari-Ankh-Ka is the most ancient form of Afrakhamitic movement and poses. (Ari = do, make; Ankh = life; Ka = soul). It literally means to make the soul come to life. Illustrations of the postures of Ari-Ankh-Ka have been found on the ancient Khamitic Temple walls. The beauty of Ari-Ankh-Ka, unlike Hatha Yoga, is that with each posture there is a specific Hesi (ancient sound). This stimulates a greater healing, oneness, inner power and balance (Maat) between the various body organs. Ari-Ankh-Ka was revived in these times by Hru Ankh Ra Semahj Se Ptah, Senur of the Temple of Ptah. Says Sen-Ur Semahj, "Ari-Ankh-Ka consciousness affirms our connectedness to the Divine, while yoga seeks to yoke to the Divine, Ari-Ankh-Ka is Hu-ka Ami Ntr — the authoritative utterance of the soul dwelling in the Divine."

An Ancient Khamitic Prayer

Offer yourself up before and after Ari-Ankh-Ka postures to the indwelling healer, the one Most High. (NTR)

AMMA SU EN PA NTR
Give yourself to the Most High.

SA-UKSU EMMENT RA EN PA NTR
Keep yourself daily for the Most High.

AU-TO AU RA MAAKETI PA HRU RA
And do it tomorrow as you do it today.

Eighteen

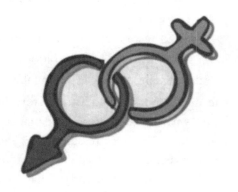

Holistic Lovemaking

Diet and Life Style in Preparation for Divine Exchange of Fluids

PREPARE YOUR MATE for clean, purified lovemaking 24 hours in advance. Take fruits so s/he will be as sweet as fruit. If you eat pork or beef, you will have a smell and taste like that of a pig or cow. Instead, eat plenty of watermelon and berries.

Partners: Be considerate. I have already discussed the negative affects of dairy products on women's reproductive organs and the direct relationship between eating dairy products and developing tumors and cysts. Men also must avoid eating dairy, as it produces unhealthy acids and mucus in the semen. A man could end up poisoning the woman he loves while exchanging body fluids during lovemaking.

The same goes for men who interact with women who regularly eat devitalized, mucus-producing foods. If her fluids (juices) are impacted with these foods, then her partner's body can become ill, particularly if he is a vegetarian, faster or fruitarian.

The lovemaking experience should be an uplifting one, not a dangerous one. Here is an herbal combination to help you prepare for lovemaking.

For men:

Burdock - cleansing and detoxing.

Use 3 tablespoons to 3 cups of water.

For women:

Red raspberry - rejuvenation of female organs.

Dandelion - healthy blood, physical strength.

Additionally, both can use alfalfa.

The diet, three to 24 hours before lovemaking, should consist of all fruits (with the exception of bananas), salads, and live vegetables and fruit juices. Freshly pressed apple, pear, pineapple, grape and papaya are all sweet nectars that help your body and temperament to be as sweet as possible. Remember that foods affect your attitude.

Also take wheatgrass. Stay away from starches, fried foods, meats, and sugar (which destroys nerves, the brain, bones, and causes stress). Take an enema, herbal laxative or Heal Thyself Colon Deblocker (3 tablespoons with lemon or lime water). Eat lots of okra, a natural laxative. Dr. Moore, may he rest in divine peace, said that okra is good for the male and female sexual organs. It acts as a rejuvenator.

Here is a bath to use in preparation for Divine Lovemaking. It can also be taken once a week to maintain a sweet, soothing disposition.

Soak individually or jointly with mate in a bath of 2-4 pounds Epsom salt, 1 cup ginger, 2 tablespoons cinnamon and 1 tablespoon nutmeg, to make a natural bubble bath. Add rose petals and enjoy for 30 minutes or more. Burn non-toxic jasmine in your bath area (hydrotherapy room), if desired. Afterwards, massage one another with sweet oils. Omit the salt if you have high blood pressure.

Heal Your Inner Environment

Don't make love if angry, mad, enraged, or in any adverse emotional state. Your state of mind will be released into your mate, who will, in turn, experience your pain. Meditate or visualize beautiful thoughts and feelings.

Some people take drugs and alcohol to make love, but it destroys the senses, poisons the blood, and invites lower (Satanic) forces into your union and distances you from the Creator.

As in all things, the Creator must be present. So, it is in lovemaking. *Note:* If you are free of drugs and alcohol and your partner is not, your pure body will take in your partner's fluids as poison. These toxins will leave the once-pure partner intoxicated, unfulfilled, unhappy and empty of spiritual food.

Heal your lover and heal thyself.

Infertility Among Women and Men

Fast as often as possible (for 7-21 days monthly for three to six months) to totally restore the reproductive organs.

Clean the colon of old, impacted waste that is probably pressing down on your organs and causing blockage.

Lay on slant board daily for 15 to 30 minutes or place face up against the wall in a 45⁰ angle with your back facing the floor. This will assist in sending an extra supply of fresh blood and oxygen to the reproductive organs and to allow for a smoother flow throughout your system.

Use Queen Afua's Clay over pelvis of both men and women for at least three to four times weekly. Cover clay with gauze overnight. The next morning shower pelvis with hot and cold water (two to three rounds).

Drink at least 12-16 ounces of carrot, beet, and scallion juice daily. Take the male and female herbal tonics listed in the Nature Cures section.

Restore Lost Fluid in Men after Lovemaking

Women, prepare and serve this formula to your love one to help prevent premature aging, sexual impotency, prostate gland blockage, and loss of hair and mental deterioration. A constant releasing of sacred fluid without replenishing will cause some or all of the above health imbalances over a period of years.

Formula: 2 tablespoons lecithin

200 mg. Vitamin E

15-30 mg. Zinc

2 ounces pumpkin seeds *(soak overnight)*

8 ounces of water

Blend together

Add raw honey or raw maple syrup, for taste.

For additional rejuvenation, take Saw Palmetto berries (2 tablespoons with 2 cups of boiling water). Steep 1 hour and drink for extra male potency. This formula can help one fight against prostrate cancer. One also can make 1 to 2 cups of ginseng to rejuvenate the prostrate.

Review Nature's Cure in chapter on men's formula, anti-prostrate cancer care.

Toward Divine Lovemaking and Conception

Two to three days prior to lovemaking, the couple should eat only fresh fruits and raw vegetables, as well as live juices. In the mornings, take the juices of 2 grapefruits and 2 oranges. Take herbal laxative or enemas daily for two to three days to unclog the reproductive organs. Take Heal Thyself Formulas I, II, and III, as well as the herbs: red raspberry for women; saw palmetto for men. Add 3 tablespoons freshly pressed ginger with each herb in water.

Fortify with:

- Breathing and exercises: 100 rounds of fire breathing together, two times a day. This will make you more sensitive to one another's touch and thoughts.

- Place legs in 45⁰ angle against the wall while lying on your back for better circulation to the sexual organs.

- Other exercises: squats, leg raises (20-30 times), sit-ups (10-30 times), pelvic lifts (four -10 times).

- While laying on back, inhale and exhale breath with each movement.

- Cleanse and energize reproductive organs. Do for two to three days. Men, apply Queen Afua's Rejuvenating Clay pack over your genitals for one hour, then shower. Women, insert clay 2 inches into the vagina with or without cotton swab; leave for one hour and wash out.

Results:

- A "sweet" vagina.
- Your body will smell and taste sweet and clean.
- More sensitive to one another's needs, thoughts and feelings.
- You will be more creative, never bored. Boredom indicates you need a great deal of cleansing and rejuvenating. The cleaner you are, the more creative and loving you are.
- No longer will you be exchanging one another's sickness.
- Orgasms will be more intense, stronger and last longer.
- You will experience the sacredness of lovemaking as a divine and blessed act.

Take a "Love Bath" before union (separately or together):

> 1 tablespoon cinnamon
> 3 tablespoons rosewater/3 teaspoons rose oil
> Natural bubble bath
> Handful of patchouli
> 1-2 pounds Dead Sea salt (for deep relaxation)
> Soak 20-30 minutes
> Soft music, small candle, fresh flowers.

Hand scrub body with lemon or grapefruit while in tub. Take shower afterwards. (*This step is optional for extra pure skin.*)

After bath:

- Dry and anoint your mate with rose water or oil. Use musk (men); sandalwood (women), or other uncut pure oil of your choice.
- Sprinkle cinnamon around the sheets (according to the late Dr. John Moore).
- Boil 1 teaspoon of cinnamon or nutmeg in a pot of water to bring a sweetness into the air of your home temple.

I recommend that you don't make love in red or black or hot pink, for it evokes only stimulation of the lower chakras. Work with the colors that are listed in handbooks to help stimulate the 4th (heart) to 7th chakras (crown, spiritual).

Don't make love haphazardly. Prepare yourself and your environment for such a divine interaction. While making love, have thoughts of giving, exchanging beauty, being respectful, being spiritual, healing and nurturing. Know that you both are a gift from the Creator to one another.

High thoughts, purified feelings and cleansed body Temples bring forth a healthy, loving and spiritually advanced child to the world through you. Preparation for conception should be three months to one year—living on a system such as described in this book.

Love taboos: Never make love when confused, angry, tired, guilty, depressed or weak, for you will poison one another through your imbalanced, devitalized fluids and weak spiritual state. When in this state, make love by long walks in the park, embraces, hand-holding and candlelit dinners to strengthen relationship and self first.

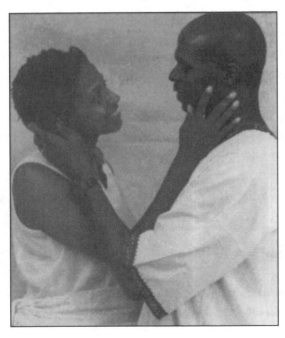

Spiritual Union

Mundane loving is not all there is. While making love, be tender, be powerful, be sweet and, oh, so gentle. Chant together. As you move, breathe in and out in sheer harmony. Whisper words of peace, joy and contentment.

During lovemaking, and, particularly, during your divine orgasm, visualize what goodness you desire for your mate and go so far as visualizing the beauty and healing you desire for the planet on which you live; for the burning fire within us is now activated and potent to move out into the Universe by way of your third eye and crown and heart chakras.

Women, say while in your lover's arms: I am a Divine Temple and I will you most Divine Love. When you enter into my temple walls, I will transform you and renew you. When you enter my gate, you will find peace, for I am pure love. You may enter, my gentle strong, king man.

Man, say while in your lover's embrace: I am the Divine DJED (Afrikan-Khamitic word meaning stability) designed for your sacred garden. As I enter my djed into your great temple walls, I come with a scepter of transformation, balance and high direction. My coming to you will bear you gifts of deep beauty and warmth, protection and peace. Allow me in, my precious queen woman, so that we may travel the galaxy as one.

And when you join together and travel through many pylons and doorways to arrive at the shore of that vast ocean of bliss, as you ride on that Great River together, an inner explosion occurs and the heavenly gates open within you, ushering a oneness upon you. Remember that moment of stillness, of splendor and tranquillity, and absorb that oneness into your life as transformative healing, for your union when pure in heart and body is a gift supreme from God to you.

Note: This level of lovemaking is almost impossible if you consume the flesh of an animal or devitalized food and drink. Men, if you persist in a destructive diet, prove your love for your mate by wearing a condom.

On Finding Your Soul Mate

To attract a divine mate, you must become divine in your state. I bear witness to countless testimonials from students and devotees of cleansing who found their soul mates. Others have healed their broken marriages by living and loving in the ways of purification.

Remember, it can happen in the twinkle of an eye or during a 21-day fast ... so fast and pray and fast and pray.

Then, one day in your divine state, a reflection of a mate will appear before your very eyes if only you would purify.

So light a pink candle and go your way and know that he/she will be coming any day.

May This Love Last Forever

The love that we exchange, let it last forever. Let love inspire, encourage, strengthen and nurture us. Let this love last forever. Let that love be within the baby that we created so beautifully; that idea that we created so brilliantly. Let love last forever, and with each love experience, let it be a lesson, a blessing, a teaching, a sharing. May this love last forever.

In Celebration of Our Men

A Love Letter

I love you, Black Man, Afrakan Man, Khamitic Man.

We, Afrakan Women, love our men.

Our unions endured through the storms, pains, pressures and hardships that kidnapped us to these shores.

Hundreds of years have gone by, yet, we still maintain our deep love for you, even when we have been separated.

In the quiet night, I called out for you.

Did you hear me?

I know you can feel me.

I love you... I've loved you from the beginning

And I will love you for all eternity.

Nothing, not even time, will stop me from loving you
My love for you is unshakable, unbreakable, unconditional and
    simply — ageless.

You are the first man, the finest man, the most regal.
All men after you, use you as the example of Manhood.
My king, scholar, leader, physician, architect, builder, lover
You are the Father, the Big Baba of the Earth.

Your Afrakan Women rise up to embrace,
    to cherish and to nurture you.
My beloved King, you have been wounded; you're bleeding
    Sound out the horns! Alert the women!
The planet is in trouble.
    The planet will not be right until you, I, we, heal.

I will patch your wounds with herbs — comfrey, red clover.
I will bathe you in hyssop.
I will anoint you with frankincense and myrrh.
I will feed you with sweet nectar.
I will help us both to heal.
So many hundreds of years have gone by.
Now, take me, rock me in your ancient arms
    and let me know all's right
With you my burden is light.
Let me rest in your mighty chest and
    become empowered by your touch.
Let me know that all is ALL RIGHT.

I need you, for your presence makes me feel like
    the burst of the sun's energy.
What joy, what peace, what pleasure, what comfort you give to
    me when you're loving me.
Oh, how my Moon loves to dance around your Sun!

Black Man, Afrakan, Khamitic Man...

You are to me the bright star that burns through the night.

Oh, how I love to touch you, and one thousand stars fill my
soul with pure ecstasy.

Your strong, loving arms open the heavens for me.

In return, I open my heart to you.

Take care of my heart.

I trust you to.

I sometimes sit and think to myself with a smile
on my face

I can see you in my mind's eye — the First Eye,

You're as sweet as brown cinnamon, as strong and as powerful
as an oak tree, as firm as a rock ...

I thank the Creator with every breath of my being
for having such a Divine and Noble Reflection.

Oh, how we love our King Man.

Can't nobody love .you—like we love you.

I love you now, I loved you then, and I will love you
for all eternity

For our love is unshakable, unbreakable, unconditional
and simply ageless.

Age less, age less... .

• • •

Write your mate a love letter, for love heals all wounds. The greatest
Medicine is Love; the greatest honor is love. Love will be showered
upon you if you give love. If love is pure and real, it will last forever.

If you are not receiving love, then you have not been giving it.
Write yourself a love letter and bring yourself fresh flowers. Speak
words of love; feel and think thoughts of love. Become love and you
will draw love unto yourself. The greatest, most perfect love is the love

we receive from the Creator. Love is a gift, a blessing. If you have it, share it. If you want it, give it.

Holistic Sharing

The Holistic Family

Traditionally, when a member of the family or tribe was ill, the whole family healed as a unit. It was never just an individual effort. Everything was done collectively. Individualism and separation from family has caused illness and need. Here are some family healing suggestions to help regain the natural, ancient, Afrikan Principles.

Suggestions for Healing the Family

All families should select one day a week for "Family Healing Day." On that day, the family does the following to prevent sickness and family disharmony. Take an herbal laxative the evening before "Family Healing Day" so that everyone purges by morning.

- Take an enema with the juice of a lemon or lime added (2 quarts of water for adults.) and a 2-4 pound salt bath. If your child is congested or suffering from a childhood dis-ease, i.e. mumps, measles or ear infections, give your child an herbal laxative or a warm water enema—if child is amenable to the idea of cleansing internally with water. (Some children, even those who are vegetarian, are clogged up; therefore, they need internal cleansing if they overdo eating too much soy meats, or whole grains and cereals. The cleaner each family member becomes; the better the communication, the sweeter the dispositions, and the more patient you will be with one another.

- Eat only live fruits and vegetables and drink 8-16 ounces each of the fresh fruit and vegetable juices.

- Participate in family morning and evening prayer, as well as shared affirmation and thanksgiving.

- Wear white or family color of choice that supports your purpose.

- Instead of watching TV, make a family video or write a family play.

- Massage one another from head to toe. Use olive oil. If you have aches and pains.

- Do a family clay and air bath, for 30 minutes — this should be healing fun!

- Have a family herbal tea party. Chat and enjoy each other. Bring fresh flowers to the home. Clean the house as a family unit.

- Say loving words to one another all day. Carry this family activity over the week in time, but always keep at least one day a week for family unity, bonding, and exchange of beauty and harmony. For without a family, there is no civilization. Include your extended family in the love process as well.

Nineteen

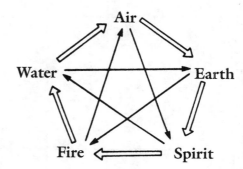

We Are
The Elements

THE BODY IS made up of all the elements that are present on the Earth. As a result, we must use those natural elements that are in nature to Heal Ourselves: air (lungs), fire (blood, reproductive organs), water (90% of the body consists of this element alone), earth (bones, teeth) and ether (spirit).

As we use the proper elements that are on earth for the healing of our body elements, then we will be in total harmony with ourselves, nature, the universe and all our relations. Refer to the following chart as you seek to balance a particular element within the body.

The planet Earth is polluted and all its people are constipated with old, impacted, undigested food and bad thoughts. Everyone has one or more of the elements in their body Temple blocked with sickness and disease. Enemas, colonics, drinking large amounts of water, fasting and herbal purges will heal all the sick, tired and over-abused body elements. Once your body is totally cleansed, then you are living the ancient quote, "Cleanliness is next to Godliness." Until your body becomes totally pure and free of all disease created by man, you will never truly be one with the Creator of the Universe. Suffering will continue to be rampant throughout the land. Follow the Element Chart to re-establish your seat in the high council of Natural Living.

Five Element Chart

Using the Angels: Earth, Air, Water, Ether (Spirit) for Natural Healing
Employ this chart to help you maintain your health balance.

	Anatomy	Foods	Colors	Physical Activities	Creative Expression
Ether	Head (Mental and spiritual center)	Honey, Fruit	White/Black, Purple	Meditation, Visualization, Instrument	Zither/Harp, Flute/String
Air	Respiratory/ Nervous system	Sprouts, Leeks, Scallions, Garlic, Radishes	White/Blue	Hatha Yoga, Tai Chi, Ari-Ankh-Ka	Singing, Flute, Air Exercise
Fire	Reproductive organs, Bloodstream	Beets, Garlic, Red grapes, Ginger, Radishes, Cayenne	Red/Orange Yellow	Jogging, Aerobics	Violin, Drums
Water	Urinary Tract, Bladder	Cucumber, Parsley, Watercress, Spirulina, Blue-green manna, Grapefruit	Blue/Green	Swimming, Sailing, Water-skiing	Piano/Flute Painting, String instruments
Earth	Bile/Bones	Carrots, Potatoes, Brown rice, turnips, whole grains	Brown, Black, Green	Biking, Walking, Jogging	Afrikan dance, Martial arts, Drums, Sculpting, Gardening

Five Element Chart

Using the Angels: Earth, Air, Water, Ether (Spirit) for Natural Healing
Employ this chart to help you maintain your health balance.

	Nature's Cure	Locations	*Colors	Herbs
Ether	Visualization Color Therapy Fasting, Crystal Healing	Botanical gardens, Mountains	White/purple	Gota Kola, Vervain, Blessed Thistle
Air	Pranayama (breathing exercise), Air Baths,	Parks, Wide open spaces	White	Apple Cider Vinegar, Eucalyptus, Camphor oil
Fire	Hot tub bath Steam Bath, Sun Baths, Sauna	New York City (Fast-paced, but be aware of burnout), Hot climate	Red (energizer), Blue (calms energy or burnout)	Gota Kola Goldenseal
Water	Colonics Baths, Enemas Nose rinses. Fasting	Oceans, Pools, Jamaica or any tropical island	Blue	Chickweed Fennel Bladderwrack
Earth	Clay packs (internal and external) Bentonite, Crystal, Healing	Beaches, Parks, Afrika	Green	Cascara Sagrada, Senna, Peppermint

Five Element Chart

Using the Angels: Earth, Air, Water, Ether (Spirit) for Natural Healing
Employ this chart to help you maintain your health balance.

	Emotional Blockage	Emotional Harmony	Physical dis-Eases
Ether	Feeling disconnected from the creator; Unable to hear your inner voice	Happiness, balance, in tune with the Creator; able to hear your inner voice	Depression, Headaches, Lack of Creativity
Air	Quick to judge; stifled and trapped; lacking in patience	Creativity, ability to move freely with ideas and concepts as well as physically and emotionally	Asthma; colds
Fire	Lack of inspiration, anger, rage	Joy; being inspired to live more fully	High blood pressure, fevers. poor blood circulation
Water	Suppressed need to cry; Feeling overwhelmed, Sadness	Harmonious, at peace	Water retention, Edema, Kidney Failure, Frequent urination
Earth	Not being able to progress, Inability to move forward; not sharing; feeling overwhelmed	Progressive, giving	Constipation, Tumors, Cysts

Twenty

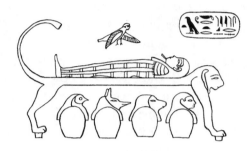

Mesu Hru— The Canopic Jars

THE TWA/ANU people of the Nile Valley were the ancestors of those who later formed the great united nation of Tawi. They preserved in their resting places a guide for those of us living in the present time. Maintenance of health precedes healing as an ideal, for in maintenance we *sustain* the balance. In healing, we seek to *restore* the balance. The ancients had a reserve of cultivated herbs and grains, to fortify them, which we do not have today.

We know the adage that prevention is better than cure. Those items that were preserved in the resting places in the Valley of the Kings and Queens are very important for us in these times. For while we may argue that some kings and queens of the nation of Tawi died at a fairly young age, the fact should be remembered that not all of us who have the information on health practice the information. As it is today, so it was then. But, the information is still available, and, if applied, can have a profound effect on the maintenance of health within the body Temple.

The Mesu Heru jars that were found are now called canopic jars. These were four jars, which contained the lungs, the liver, the small intestines and combined into one jar the stomach and large intestines. Our early ancestors (another way of saying "we" in our more ancient phases) placed as Guardians on the lids of the four jars, a Baboon, Falcon, a Jackal and a Man.

In the resting place of the Boy King, ATEN-RA-TUT-ANKH, called King Tut, we find what we believe here at the Shrine/Temple of Ptah to be a revelation that we, of the present time, can be guided by. This revelation is of great importance because that young King's resting place was the only one found intact in modern times. The majority of what was found is still preserved. Revelation tells us that the preservation of this vital resting place of King Tut is for us, his brothers and sisters in these times, a time capsule that we can study and use for the reclamation of our Khamitic heritage and legacy. It is why I say health is a High Science. A reclamation of this legacy must begin, first of all with the recognition that we have become a sick people and our first business is to heal ourselves.

We cannot seek to change the condition by which we've become surrounded—unless we begin with self. We are off-track because of the ingestion of the wrong diet imposed upon us by foreigners. And so that's the reason why this information was all the more important for the initiate. It served to preserve him/her in a state of health in order to combat the conditions that were pressing in on us then, as they are now.

The jar that contained the lungs in King Tut's resting place was positioned on the eastern wall of the tomb. So to us, this is a revelation that the east is a place of beginning as we go in a clockwise position. On the eastern wall is represented the guardian *Hapi* and the face used to cover this jar was the cynocephalus baboon (see Fig. 1). This was one of the so-called sacred baboons, associated with the Ntr *Tehuti*, who is the guardian of letters, of intelligence, and the keeper of time.

In the beginning, we said that these heads were chosen because each head indicated that principle for which the organ was created and by which it can be maintained. The baboon urinates every hour on the hour, so its head was used to be an archetype of periodicity. This brings to mind that our breaths are likewise numbered. We must in cadence practice breathing, which is called in yoga *pranayama*. Hapi's color is black to indigo. Hapi means dual, vital force—inhalation and exhalation. We may choose licorice, comfrey root and other herbs to maintain this organ. Those herbs that will support the element of air are the herbs that we should ingest for the maintenance of this guardian. A guardian is a servant, like an angel, and as such, in the Afrakan context, must be fed its proper food, i.e. the herbs mentioned previously.

As we now come to the south, we have *Qbsenuf,* the guardian of the small intestine (Fig. 2). Qbsenuf's animal is the falcon. We know that the blood consumes its food through the walls of the small intestine and, thus, the nourishment is transferred along this passage. The nourishing chyle is offered to the blood as sustenance and this then aids the warrior within to conduct the battle against dis-ease. Chyle is the substance which nourishes the blood; it is made from chyme. The falcon is commonly referred to as a warrior bird, and it has always been the perennial symbol of the Khamitic royalty of Tawi. The keen vision of the bird also is very well known. Among hunters, it is used in the art of what they call falconry. Hence, our ancestors chose this bird to indicate the spiritual energy that comes from the foods fed to the intestine; and the spirit of speed, of deep, piercing sight and ascension to spiritual heights, which the falcon exemplifies.

The color for the guardian of the small intestine is white, and as such, the foods are garlic, ginger, etc. It is, at this point, that the watery chyle is literally wrung out through 26 feet of intestines. This guardian's element is water and it would require us to consume water to help to maintain the fluidity and peristaltic activity of this organ.

To the west, the guardian has the face of a man and he has the name *Amset* (Fig. 3). Amset is the guardian of the liver. His color is green, which refers to the bile and also to its opposite (yellow) when the liver is vexed. The yellow indicates jaundice.

This is one of the most important organs in the maintenance of the cleanliness of the blood and so it must be fed its proper food, such as chlorophyll, peppermint, aloes, etc. to be maintained in a state of calm. The liver is known to register the emotions of the individual and so the face of a man was put on it because in the face we can read the condition of one's liver. A calm face would indicate that the liver is, likewise, calm, and is being properly maintained. It is on the face that the emotions are mainly registered, eg. alcohol, vexes the liver and depresses the spirit. This guardian rules the element earth.

The jar with the head of a jackal represents *Tuamutf* and the cardinal point, north. Tuamutf presides over the functions of the stomach and large intestines. The food in the stomach is in a partial state of digestion. We should say that it begins at the very thought of eating because the salivary glands begin to do their work in preparation for the breakdown of food in the mouth. The stomach, the pouch at the bottom, catches what we ingest.

In the stomach, the food goes through the most pronounced function of digestion because it's here that the digestive juices (enzymes, acids and alkalies) produce the chyme, which the small intestines assimilates. It's also a place where further digestion takes place. *So, it is important that peristaltic action of this organ be kept in tone with fire foods where we find the color red ruling.* The foods that have blossoms and seeds of red are particularly good for maintaining the health of this organ. Cayenne pepper, sorrel, watermelon, beets (preferably when young to lessen the amount of starch), and other foods that have red in them will aid in the maintenance of the fires of Tuamutf.

Hapi — is the name of the river that we call the Nile today. It is associated with the bull because the river, in its inundation, was seen as a bull — strong, vital and regenerative. Hapi is also the name of the constellation, which we now know as Aquarius. Hapi is the Khamitic name and sound. In this age, the element of air rules and Hapi is the ruler of the lungs. We are bombarded in this age by the impurities in the air, and so it is important that we feed detoxifying foods to Hapi to reduce the damage of modern life.

Qbsenuf — the name means "he refreshes his brethren." The refreshment is the nourishment of the foods going to the blood stream. The name envelopes this principle in action.

Amset — the very name means green. This is the seed of nourishment. It is also the place where the youth of the body can be maintained. We target purifying foods for the liver. Bitter foods correspond with the substance produced by the liver.

Tuamutf — means "to praise." "Mut" means mother, "F" is the personal pronoun "His." It translates to He praises his mother, the fire from the energy that comes from the Divine Mother is the topsoil, which delivers the vegetation that we take in for the nourishment of the body. The stomach literally praises this Divine principle.

Sound also is very important and vital to the maintenance of these organs. These names, as with man when uttered, tone the respective organs.

MESU HRU
(The Canopic Jars)

FIGURE 1   FIGURE 2   FIGURE 3   FIGURE 4

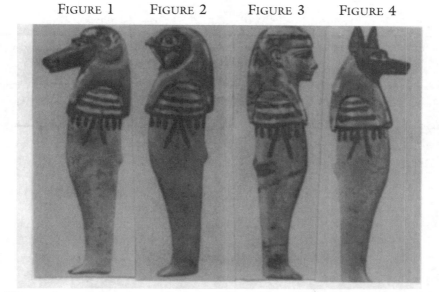

The male guardians are called the MESU HRU (children of Hru). The female nurturers are MUTU EM MESU HRU (mothers of the children of Hru). These female nurturers who stand guard over the male Neteru are Nebt Het over Hapi, Serkhet over Qbsenuf, Ast over Amset, and Net over Tuamutf. Feed them with herbs and evoke their names for "toning" of the organ with sound vibrations. HRU (You) are the immaculate Divine Child born of the union of AST (Mother principle) and ASR (Father principle).

HRU ANKH RA SEMAHJ SE PTAH

THE KHAMITIC ELEMENT CHART FOR HARMONY

Neteru	Figure 1	Figure 2	Figure 3	Figure 4
Direction	East	South	West	North
Male *Guardian* Female	Hapi Nebt Het	Qbsenuf Serkhet	Amset Ast	Tua-mut-f Nt
Organs Guardian Task	Lungs Breath-regulation	Sm. intestine Absorption	Liver Blood-purification	Lg. intestine /stomach Digestion/
Color	Black/indigo	White	Green/yellow	Red
Herbs	Licorice comfrey ...	Garlic, ginger, etc.	Mints, etc.	Cayenne etc.
Element	Air	Water	Earth	Fire

Twenty-One

Spirituality

*The Ankh is the ancient Afrakan symbol for
eternal life and spiritual, physical harmony.*

A Cleansed Body Temple Is A Prayerful One. So Fast And Pray!

CULTIVATE TRANQUILITY, harmony, love and health by letting life be a
prayer. Let your every word, movement, thought, your comings and
goings, your joy, your sadness, your inhalation and exhalation, your
every breath, your work and play be prayer. For in that continuous
prayer, you shall dwell in heaven on earth. Your body Temple will
become one of pure light and love, a perfect reflection of the Creator.
When you live in this natural, divine way, a golden stream of blessings
continually flows your way. There, no disease can be found; only
health, wealth and happiness abound. So fast and pray. Pray and fast
misery away.

As you *prepare* your juices, let it be a prayer. As you *drink* your
juices and herbs, allow them to flow through as you fill up with light
and love. With each drink, see your aura improve. See yourself become
illuminated, moving beyond the Earth's toxic plane. See that sacred
nectar transform you.

As you rise at dawn and rest at sunset, as you cleanse your home,
your temple, your sanctuary, let it be an act of worship. As you sit,
stand, walk, let your prayers come through.

As you "be" love, as you make love, offer it all up in prayer. Then and only then will all that you do and say be protected from all harms, all hurt, and all darkness. There is no darkness in prayer, only the light of the Creator. So fast and pray.

Devotion to Purification as a Spiritual Path

When you are cleansed or are a "Devotee/Initiate of Purification," you no longer resort to destructive behavior, such as the use of self-abusive elements, i.e., alcohol, drugs, tobacco, gossiping or complaining. You follow the "26 Laws for Devotees of Purification as a Spiritual Path." Practice the following:

Exercise, take walks, salt baths, or showers.

Drink glasses of warm water or a Heal Thyself Nutritional Formula with juice.

Pray or meditate daily or weekly.

Fast on fruit and vegetable juices.

Give thanks and praise.

Each time you choose this progressive response/action, you climb higher and higher into your spiritual and physical self-healing. It cannot be said enough. A Devotee of Purification is one who will purify at all costs. Regardless of what is going on in their lives, they will cleanse.

If upset, take a bath.

If you have lost your mate, cleanse your home.

If lacking money, wear green, light a green candle and pray.

If confused, take gota kola and do shoulder or headstands.

26 Laws For Devotees of Purification

1. Fast and purify for all seasons, conditions and circumstances.
2. Pray daily as the 3 cycles of the sun are being ushered in.
3. Maintain clean thoughts, heart, and feelings at all costs.
4. Fast and purify on your personal Holy Day and your community's Holy Day.
5. Live by the *Heal Thyself* text.
6. Women: fast during your menses or eat only live foods. Men:

during your mate's menses, fast and pray with her for Divine harmony and a cleansing of the relationship.

7. Free yourself from disease of the body Temple, heart, and mind.

8. Become a vegetarian, fruitarian, or 'liquitarian.'

9. Do not use drugs, alcohol or engage in out-of-season lovemaking.

10. Follow the Dietary Timetable that is ruled by the Sun.

11. Begin a fast or purification ritual with every seasonal change, with every new moon (for 24-36 hours) to affirm new dreams and prayers.

12. Silently meditate every full moon period. Take green juices and rejuvenating herbs during this time for inner peace and balance (Maat).

13. Pray daily for universal peace and purification for yourself, for family, nation and world.

14. The clothing you wear must reflect the beauty and harmony seen in nature and the oneness with the Holy Spirit. Use color charts to assist your choice as to what you want to express to the world and attract or repel from you.

15. Support all those in their healing who request your assistance in some way, big or small. In this way, you support yourself.

16. Use the four elements to heal yourself daily.

17. Become active in spiritual and community work of your choice.

18. Give selfless service/aid to someone less fortunate than yourself as often as possible, or, at least, during every new moon period.

19. Fast every new moon and full moon on vegetable and fruit juices, and water. This fast I've done with a guru friend from the Hare Krishna Temple. I don't advise it unless you are guided by a profound spiritual devotee.

20. Show love, give love, and appreciate love with and from your birth family, extended family and all your relations, including the spiritual family you adopt.

21. Be the first to ask for forgiveness; be the first to forgive.

22. As a city dweller, go to rest in parks, or by the ocean to recharge your spiritual and physical self.

23. As a country dweller, be blessed to be able to visit nature daily.

24. Let your home be your Temple, your sanctuary. Purify it daily with water, frankincense and myrrh, sage and cedar.

25. Recognize cleansing as a spiritual practice our ancient ancestors used as a rite of passage for initiates into higher understanding and the Mysteries.

26. Listen inwardly for total guidance every step of the way.

Daily Spiritual Purification Discipline

1. 6:00 a.m. Sun Rise
   Recite Water Prayer (see *Hydrotherapy*) while taking shower or bath. Dry your body and put on white attire before going into prayer.

2. Sit on chair or pillow. (*Be sure to open a window in the room in which you're praying.*) Perform the Breath of Life Exercises:

   25-100 Cooling Breaths for night.

   100 Fire Breaths (*500 Fire Breaths for work*).

   Sing or chant/spiritual songs or chant the universal sound "OM." "ANKH, using the high-pitched, nasal tone in Asar Aset song."

3. Read a passage from your personal spiritual book.
   For example:
   Hu Sia
   Holy Bible
   Book of Coming Forth To Day from Night
   (misnomered *The Egyptian Book of the Dead*)
   The Upanishads
   Essene Gospel of Peace
   Holy Qu'ran
   Kahlil Gibran's *The Prophet*, etc.

4. Activities of Prayer Session
   (a) Thanksgiving
   (b) Prayers
   (c) Forgiving
   (d) Affirmations

(e) Seeing the Future As You'd like It to Be

(f) Evaluation of Day

5. Song/Chant—to reinforce the "fasting and chanting"

   After chanting, go into meditation for 5, 30 or 60 minutes.

6. *Become the Ocean of Life or the Song of the Day*

   Set up a simple altar comprising:

   • one glass of water to absorb negative vibrations
   • a spiritual book
   • crystals to purify and charge the area
   • pyramid (*optional*)
   • fresh flowers
   • picture of spiritual teacher in this world or the spirit world (*your ancestors*)
   • cloth to cover low, prayer table
   • candle 15 hours or 7 days (*Place candle in a glass bowl.*)
   • Burn non-toxic incense of jasmine or frankincense and myrrh with charcoal to purify the home.

A FASTING POEM

Confessions of a Low-Vibration Junkie

Day breaks!
Got the Shakes!
Mind slipping...
Nose dripping
Body aches
    I feel real bad, like the flu,
I got the detoxification blues ...
Got an attitude. Feeling bad.
Want some fried chicken, Mad...
    You see, you see
    "My Jones is coming down on me."
Why won't these toxins let me be?

I want to be free, free, free.
Ringgggg, ring, ring — "Yes, Queen Afua, I know;
   take two enemas and call you in the morning."

    Bacon, eggs, cheese on toast.
Mmmmmmmmmmmmm, yea, yea ... No!
It's really puss on toast
Mucus on toast.
    The Last Poets
That doesn't sound good
I'll eat/drink what I should
Yea, some Lecithin, Spirulina, TwinLab,
And, of course, the carrot-beet.
Mmmmmm, yea that should put me on my feet.
Now, I'm ready to hit the street ...
    But, the situation remains ...
and it's plain ...
and it be ...
My Jones, my Jones is coming down on me.

Roger Moore,
A 21-day Faster

Twenty-Two

Heal Thyself Formulas for Fasting and Healing

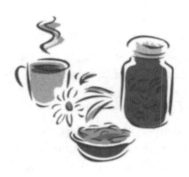

YOUR GENERAL NUTRITIONAL supplement is spirulina or wheatgrass (powdered), or a more potent 1-2 ounces of liquid wheatgrass. Take 1 tablespoon of spirulina, wheatgrass or Queen Afua's Super Nutritional Formula I three times daily with juice. If you have a chronic disease, for intense rejuvenating, take 1 tablespoon of both spirulina and wheatgrass. If you feel nausea after taking this combination, reduce the amount by one-half. Once your body is cleansed, you will be able to handle the chlorophyll, and you will be able to take larger amounts of green drinks (as much as up to 2-3 tablespoons of either, or 2 ounces of fresh-pressed wheatgrass).

Take Vitamin C, in the form of lemon, lime, grapefruit, rosehips tea, cayenne pepper, or Vitamin C 500-1000 mg., twice a day, up to three times a day when fasting. Heal Thyself health products are geared towards achieving health through nutritional fasting and natural healing.

Queen Afua's Super Nutritional Formula I

The Super Nutritional Formula of wheatgrass and spirulina is an almost complete food. The addition of psyllium aids in the elimination of old, impacted waste trapped in the colon.

Formula I contains:

Vitamins A, B_1, B_2 -Folic Acid, B_3 -Chlorine, B_5 -Inositol, B_6, B_{12}, B_{17} (the entire Vitamin B complex), Vitamins C (ascorbic acid), E, F, K, Potassium, Copper, Iron, Calcium, Chromium, Magnesium, Manganese, Sodium, Zinc, Phosphorus, Selenium, Silicon, Cobalt, Sulfur, and trace minerals.

Vitamin K helps prevents kidney stones; it also helps one to digest calcium and protein.

To Prepare Formula I:

Blend and drink promptly 1-2 tablespoons of Formula I with fresh fruit or vegetable juice 2-3 times daily.

Take additional B Vitamins for anti-stress.

If you have skin problems or a nervous condition, take 2 tablespoons of chlorophyll in addition to B vitamins. If problem persists after a week or two, add TwinLab yeast without the whey (liquid form from 15-50 mg.)

For best results, contact a nutritionist, a naturopath, an herbalist or holistic health consultant to give you the personal guidance you may need.

Use the above information, as well as all the information in my book, as a general guide.

Queen Afua's Master Herbal Formula II

The Master Formula II contains: 13 powerful herbs designed to strengthen and cleanse every system within the body Temple. (This formula builds a strong body Temple).

Ingredients include:

1. *Gota Kola* - A brain food and stimulant.
2. *Comfrey* - for cleansing, healing and knitting of bones, internally and externally. This herb food is excellent for male and female productive organs, as well as bladder and kidney toning. Comfrey is high in calcium.
3. *Alfalfa* - builds and strengthens. It contains Vitamin A, E, K,

B, helps to fight alcoholism and stress, and builds the immune system. Alfalfa contains protein, phosphorus, iron, potassium, chlorine, silicon, magnesium and sodium, and has within it 8 enzymes that promote chemical reactions enabling food to assimilate within the body.

4. *Echinacea* - a blood cleanser and antiseptic, reduces glandular swelling.

5. *Blessed Thistle* - strengthens the heart, liver, lungs, and kidneys.

6. *Red Clover* - a blood purifier and an anti-cancer herb, soothes the nerves and rejuvenates the gall bladder.

7. *Cascara Sagrada* - relieves chronic constipation; is an intestinal tonic and assists in cleansing the liver.

8. *Mullein* - valuable in asthma and lung afflictions, aids in calming the nerves and in eliminating ulcers and tumors.

9. *Chickweed* - is excellent for weight loss. It aids inflamed eyes and skin disease. (The late Dr. John Moore also recommended this herb to help burn excess fat.)

10. *Dandelion* - purifies and helps to neutralize the acids in the blood. It eliminates anemia, and aids in skin disease, such as jaundice and eczema. It is useful in relieving kidney conditions.

11. *Ginger* - increases circulation and expel mucus congestion.

12. *Chaparral* - an anti-cancer herb.

13. *Fenugreek* - clears mucus from the bronchial passages and has a healing effect on the bowels.

To Prepare Formula II:

Boil 4-5 cups of purified or distilled water.

Turn off boiling water and add 4-5 teaspoons of herbal mixture (Formula II).

Allow it to steep overnight. Strain in the morning. (Use the leftover herbs in a bath and soak.) Do not reheat or refrigerate. Drink from morning to 12 p.m. (High Noon) for freshness and potency. Take 5-7 times a week.

Note: Vitamin D, T and U, although not in Super Nutritional Formula

I, are contained in the Master Herbal Formula II. Vitamin P (Bioflavonoids) can be acquired from the white, inner skin of lemons, oranges, and grapefruit. Iodine can be obtained from kelp, watercress and artichokes, to name a few sources.

Formula III — Colon Deblocker

The Colon Deblocker contains three potent cleansing oils to lubricate and detoxify old, impacted waste from the colon.

Ingredients: Castor oil, cold-pressed olive oil and Vitamin E.

To prepare Formula III:

Take 2-3 tablespoons of Formula III daily with the juice of 1 lime or lemon, or with Kidney-Liver Flush, first thing in the morning. Take every other day when fasting. Take 1-2 times a week while on the Natural Living Program.

* * *

I've met a woman on the Path of Purification a healer whose gift was the power of Love and Forgiveness. Her name is Queen Esther.

Our vision of Healing is one; we are inseparable, bounded by joy. We had everything in common; the love of art, dance, our children, vegetarian life style and the love and appreciation of our culture.

One early afternoon, as we sat at the kitchen table, feverously talking and laughing about life, just sharing our stories. Silence came over us. We agreed to become blood sisters. We performed the ritual of sister to sister, like little, innocent girls; we broke open the skin of our fourth finger with a needle, joined fingers and touched one another's blood. We became sisters and vowed to be there for each other.

As time went on, Queen Esther became a part of Heal Thyself staff team in 1987. She was a joy to work with; rather she was administering colonics or rendering wellness consultations, giving dance classes or natural beauty treatments. Love and joy poured out from her to all those she met. Divine spirit guided me to ask Queen Esther to share her heart on Healing with you within the *Heal Thyself* text.

A Word To The Healers

Healing was very sacred work in ancient times and is still sacred today. The healing arts were for priests and priestesses, medicine men and women, "bush" doctors and other people who were respected for their knowledge in the sacred mystery systems.

However, when these three major aspects of the body, mental, physical and spiritual are out of order or alignment, there is then a malfunctioning and the individual needs healing, realignment and rejuvenation. When any of these areas are out of order, they affect the other areas.

Oftentimes when people go to the hospitals for treatment, the doctors focus on their physical ailments and never look into the mental or spiritual discord, which, perhaps, could be the root of the illness in the first place. When there is some mental disorder detected, patients are sent to psychiatrists, psychologists and others who focus on mental disorders. Patients are sent to different specialists who handle only an aspect of the person's problem(s). As a result, people may be left feeling disoriented or dissected.

Healing, on the other hand, is meant to bring the person into a state of oneness, order and balance; to bring all of the different aspects together in harmony. True healing comes from the Creator, and, thus, when we are living the natural laws and in tune to the Creator and the natural laws of the universe, we are healed. We are at peace within our bodies.

Medical doctors take oaths to execute the best service they can with the knowledge that they have acquired. It also is the responsibility of the healers to be good examples of what a healed person is—before they can begin healing treatments on others.

We realize that the oath of healers must include being clear, clean vessels so that the Creator can work through us to help to heal others.

Our first responsibility is to heal ourselves so that we may become shining examples of positivity, of intelligence, of love, of cleanliness, of strength, of kindness, of right thinking and right action, for these are aspects of the Most High that are associated with true healing.

I remember times in the past when I hesitated going for spiritual readings or healing because the practitioners themselves did not look healthy or happy, positive or pure. This made me feel that whatever reading I got could not be a higher vibration than the person delivering the information. In relation to this, no matter how wonderful a beautician may style your hair, the vibration of the beautician is still upon your head.

This message to healers emphasizes that no matter how long you have been practicing your particular craft, all that is not of the Most High will be exposed eventually, for "no lie can last forever."

Total healing consists of 360º of healing — in body, mind, and spirit. Until the healers understands this, and lives this in their own lives, they will never be able to heal their clients, and they will always feel that something, in their lives, is missing. The healing will still be incomplete.

Let us surrender ourselves to the Master Healer and ask to be forgiven for our shortcomings. Let us humble ourselves so that we may be truly uplifted into pure light. We will, thereby, walk with a glow and radiance around us. We will be holy in spirit so that we may be true servants of the Most High. We wish to be used to help heal our people and this planet, in truth, and in righteousness, in the name of the Most High.

Queen Esther
A Devotee and Guide of Purification

My Eldest—A Devotee of Purification

In 1992, Supa Nova, my eldest son, went to live down South in Greenboro, North Carolina with his aunt. While away, he went through an amazing transformation. He began to meditate regularly and drink large amounts of green juice daily. In addition, although Supa Nova was 17 years of age and in high school, he spent much of his time on the campus of North Carolina A&T University, giving spiritual readings to some of the college students. While there, we spoke a great deal on the phone about spiritual matters, relationships and personal healing. We could go on sometimes for hours, laughing, conversing and praying. The year that Supa Nova was away he transformed from a *vegetarian* to a *chlorophyllion*.

Upon his return home to Brooklyn, New York, at the age of 18, and after he graduated from high school, in the summer of 1993, Supa Nova came into the Heal Thyself Center as a staff member. I noticed Supa Nova carried a gallon jug of distilled water and liquid chlorophyll, cranberry juice or fresh green juice into work, to drink throughout the day. He also would carry to work a large container of a green, leafy salad to eat for lunch. At the end of the summer, he began to speak of a revelation. I felt this was profound. The following is what Supa Nova shared with me as he proclaimed, "Mom," on a hot, summer afternoon, "I'm a hip-hop Celestial, Khametic, Nubian, Chlorophyllion…" I'll let him tell the rest.

We Are What We Eat

HOTEP (PEACE) AND blessings. My name is Supa Nova Slom, son of Queen Afua. I was born and raised a vegetarian from my mother's womb. It was challenging because there were other young people who were not vegetarians, so I had to struggle to maintain my vegetarianism among my peers who were into junk foods and eating meats and so forth. I did pretty good coming up to maintain. The basic things that were taught to me by my mother were, "The body is a living church;

a living house. If you put death into your body, son," she'd say, "then your body will reflect death. If you put living, whole foods, foods that bring life to your living body, it will generate better health." It made sense when I was small and that's what I told my peers. They laughed at me because I ate natural, edible flowers and a lot of greens, but some of my peers who laughed at me, some of them now have early stages of prostrate cancer. Some of them have heavy asthma; some have osteoporosis. These are some of the diseases that are created from eating toxic foods. When I grew older, I met other vegetarians who were born as meat-eaters, but were sick and tired of being sick and tired, and decided to make the transition to a whole foods life style to save their lives, by using nature's best foods to 'heal thyself' and maintain optimum health.

Naturally, the kind of vegetarian I was raised to be was one who ate a great deal of vegetables because that's what vegetarianism is in my definition and what I've understood it to be. A vegetarian is one who eats more vegetables. Terrain refers to being of the land. If I'm eating vegetables I'm being, I'm eating, I'm consuming vegetables of the terrain. But, as I go into many wholistic supermarkets that sell organic foods and vegetarian foods, everybody's shopping cart doesn't reflect vegetarian living at least to the definition I follow. Everybody's cart has soy-this and soy-that, soy protein, soya milk, etc. These are good foods, but there are little to no vegetables in these carts. I mean, these are the ways of the general population, which is into vegetarianism. When I go to different health food stores in my hometown of Brooklyn, New York, the young people and the older people there alike, they have the whole grains in their carts; they have the nuts in their carts, but not that many vegetables. And I'm thinking because of the way that I was raised—if you're a vegetarian, the majority of your consumption should be of vegetables. It just makes sense to me.

As the media gets into this vegetarianism and it's becoming more vogue in diverse circles and among many entertainers, you can go into our Black communities, and find soy milk and tofu, which is now more available than it was when I was coming up. Now, that I'm a young man of 25, I can find a few of these natural foods accessible in my neighborhood. Generally, people's perception of vegetarianism centers in the consumption of starchy foods, soy protein, soy chicken, and soy meat, texturized soya proteins, which looks like beef or tastes a little like chicken. These are meat substitutes for those who are striving to overcome a meat diet.

These soya products are good when you're making a transition from being a carnivore (flesh-eater) to a herbivore (vegetarian). A lot of vegetarians are getting stuck in the transition, coming from the life style of eating meat or a flesh diet and are moving into a starch-substitute diet. The starch is a substitute because they still feel the need to consume foods that are heavy and filling. They don't want to just eat salads because it's not heavy enough. So, due to my observations, I realize that they are *starchetarians*. They're not vegetarians because a vegetarian would be consuming a majority of vegetables; anywhere between 90 percent to a full 100 percent of vegetables. A starchetarian would be consuming anywhere between 90 percent to 100 percent of starches.

In my observation, the majority of the people in the health food stores are starchetarians. They're wholistic starchetarians. I wouldn't call them vegetarians because when you look in their shopping carts the majority of the foods are starches, grains, whole nuts, breads and pastas, cereals, brown rice, and soy products.

Most mainstream vegetarians eat little to minimum amounts of vegetables, and if they eat vegetables, it's not live, fresh vegetables. It's over-cooked vegetables, which have minimal nutrients left. This is good for someone who's on a transition from a heavy, flesh diet moving into the wholistic, live diet. There's a new terminology out now called vegan, the vegan vegetarian. That means you don't eat any animal bi-products; you're strictly a vegetarian. But still, the vegan is associated with the general vegetarian because they still eat a majority of starches.

Now, I'm not saying anything is wrong with eating starches. All I'm saying is that we need to be clear on the precise definition of our consumption, the art of consumption, and what we are consuming. There are different types of tarians. A liquitarian is when you just have everything liquid. Say you have just liquids of fresh fruit juices, fresh vegetable juices and herbal teas and herbal tonics. That is a liquitarian. A fruitarian is someone who consumes 90 percent to 100 percent of just fruits. (*Queen Afua does not recommend a fruitarian diet in this day and age due to the high toxic level of our planet.*) The 90 percent basic is the fruit and 10 percent could be your greens and, maybe, starches and vegetables. A vegetarian, a true vegetarian, would be consuming 90 percent to 100 percent of strictly vegetables and 10 percent would be fruits, grains, whole nuts, but the majority of the consumption would be chlorophylic foods—green, leafy foods.

Based on my cultivation, the majority of my consumption was vegetables. It was not starches. My brother and sister, Sherease Torain and Ali Torain, also were raised vegetarians like me, but they were more into eating starches. They ate soy-this and soy-that and not an abundance of vegetables. They were my earliest observation of starchetarians with a 30 percent vegetable consumption.

Most vegetarians are not aware that they are starchetarians. They're consuming a vast amount of starches and they call themselves vegetarians. To clarify and avoid confusion, I have to distinguish myself from them and let it be known that I'm a *chlorophyllion*. A *chlorophyllion* is Supa Nova Slom's true definition for a true vegetarian, not a vegan and not a vegetarian—the true vegetarian. A *chlorophyllion* will consume 90 percent to 100 percent full capacity of chlorophylic foods—because with chlorophylic foods like your kale, spinach, your broccoli, chard, and all your green, leafy vegetables, including parsley, barley and wheatgrass, you have a rich capacity for protein and calcium. So, I get all of my protein and my needed calcium from the kale. Kale, out of all the green leaves, has the highest potency of calcium, so does wheatgrass, which rejuvenates the cells, boosts the immune system, helps digestion and strengthens the bones. So, with that being said, that's what makes Supa Nova Slom a *chlorophyllion*.

Chlorophyll is liquid oxygen to the body Temple. That's the difference between a 'commercial' vegan/vegetarian and a *chlorophyllion*. A modern vegetarian is really a *starchetarian*. They don't realize this, but I'm telling you right now. If you're consuming 90 percent to 100 percent mainly starches, you are a starchetarian, period. If you're consuming a majority of vegetables, you are a *true* vegetarian, or *chlorophyllion*. What we do with the tarians like a true vegetarian/chlorophyllion, starchetarian, fruitarian, we give a 10 percent waiver because the majority of your consumption would be anywhere between 80 percent or 90 percent of what you're consuming.

We want to go into one more point in closing on the art of consumption. When we deal with the physical body Temple, the body Temple is the house given by the Creator, the One Most High. The Mother/Father Creator gave our Temples to us. It is living. If we put foods of death into the Divine Temple, our body Temple becomes devitalized and disintegration sets in.

Why should the Creative Force, external/internal, come bless us when we don't even take care of the Temple, church that we were blessed to maintain. In review, remember that the *chlorophyllion* is the true vegetarian: 90 percent to 100 percent of chlorophylic foods.

I remain Supa Nova Slom, representing the Hip-Hop Generation, the medium of balance and the Khamitic Generation, and resurrection.

Hotep and Blessings

Supa Nova

P.S. Stock up on the Heal Thyself Green Life Formula I to maintain a vital *chlorophyllion* life style, and to my Khamatic Nubians, Baba Heru says, "In order to resurrect the spirit of Ausar, the father of vegetation from within, the initiate must consume the greens!" *

I've analyzed and reflected on Supa Nova's findings and have come up with the following conclusion. Those who are starchetarians, who consume large amounts of starchy foods on a daily basis, I find their temperaments are for the most part, possessive or suppressive, quick to anger or fearful, and, at times, they appear mentally hostile to others through the medium of gossip. On a physical level, a starchetarian may show signs of stagnation in their relationships and careers. They may be constipated, have tumors or sinus conditions, i.e. allergy, hay fever, colds or they may experience loss of hearing, poor memory, etc. due to clogged arteries, sluggish blood and the lack of oxygen contained in a starch-filled body Temple.

I find, on the other hand, generally those who are highly evolved vegetarians or *chlorophyllions* are more loving, compassionate and tolerant of people's differences and also are usually more spiritually, mentally, and physically electrifying.

My son's revelation has greatly inspired me to grow into a live-food chlorophyllion. Through trial and error, I have evolved. I have observed over the last 8 years of my personal transformation, that my temperament has changed considerably. People just don't get me worked up and upset anymore; I feel so joyous and free in my spirit. I'm always busy laughing, smiling and creating new and exciting healing projects. My inner gateways have flung open. My heart center is flowing; I'm in a constant state of gratitude, forgiveness, tolerance and compassion.

Regardless of people's states of consciousness, I dwell in a space of Divine loving detachment. I look at life from a healer's perspective. I understand that everyone is going through their own evolutionary stages and varied levels of healing and awakening, or stages and levels of stagnation and dis-ease. Still, all are seeking liberation on some level. As I drink my green juices and eat my green salads and sprouts, I can accept and support everyone growing at their own pace and in their own time.

As my cells recharge and my body Temple reconnects through this chlorophyllion way of life, inner peace radiates through me in the midst of life's storms and sun-rises. I'm steady as the roots of kale, broccoli and chard. I'm feeling the wings of MAAT and my heart is as light as her feathers, and this, for me, is amazing grace. Because I've been devoted to the life of a chlorophyllion. I've been blessed to have been given the temperament of a healer, and I am healing myself with every green leaf I consume, for inside of that leaf, the Most High healing light dwells.

In conclusion, I've found that the more chlorophyllic foods you consume, i.e. green vegetable juices, wheatgrass, sprouts, alfalfa, dandelion, dark green salads, etc. the purer your blood, the less starch you ingest, the less dis-eased, the more forgiving, loving, serene and strong you will be. While living a chlorophyllion life style, no matter how negative a situation or person is toward you due to their flesh or starch life style, you, as a chlorophyllion, will grow vigorously beyond and against all odds. As you embrace your Green Life, you will experience Divine protection. Negative people and situations will fall from you and positive people and situations will seek you out. Remember "water seeks its own level." So, in your transition, don't be angry about your past or present condition; learn from it. Live the miracle, "eat the green blades of the field," and experience Khepera (transformation) and become pure Ra (light). Continue to purify your karma and pay up your spiritual debt, your shai. Through the drinking of green juices, green foods, pure water and prayers, you can't help but attract the absolute best from Creation.

Thank you Supa Nova, for raising your mother's frequency. You are my young Heru, my Hero. May the light of NTR, the Divine, keep shining through you and all your revelations.

Queen Afua's Eight Greatest Lessons

The Eight Greatest Lessons that I've gathered and shared, in my 30 year walk on the Heal Thyself Path of Purification, are as follows:

1. *Be Patient*

> One day, you do well on your Natural Living Life Style; the next day, you succumb to toxic, old habits. Practice right now being patient with yourself, for it will take time to break old, poisonous patterns that comforted you, in the past. Be persistent; you will be victorious in your wellness transformation. Just be patient.

2. *Healing Never Ends*

> So you've reached your wellness goal; then, all of a sudden another fault, weakness or challenge surfaces. You're at it again. Striving to heal yourself, never giving up on yourself. What a blessing to clean up your life in stages. You're unfolding like a lotus, constantly healing your life, for healing never ends.

3. *Don't Be Afraid of Change*

> You're seeking a healing miracle. Yes, a healthier way of life. Allow yourself to move beyond your fears, pass your blocks, embrace the change, hold tight to Natural Living—for transformation is in sight.

4. *Keep on Keeping on*

> If you fall off your Wellness journey, reflect on what caused the fall. Don't give up the light. You've slipped or crashed and ate junk food, or fast food to somehow ease your life trip. You consumed, dined, or slept with death, to get relief; it was an illusion. You feel worse. It's okay; just pick yourself up, right now. Today! Make it happen once again. You're surely worth the rise, so shine bright. Just keep on keeping on, for inside you is the light.

5. *Create An Inner World of Harmony*

In seeking a place of refuge, we travel here, there and everywhere. Be still; Go within. Create an inner environment that will evoke comfort, harmony and serenity. Work to cultivate this environment from sunrise to sunset, from deep inside yourself. Purify and rejuvenate your world; become a garden of true, everlasting beauty that will always comfort and soothe you wholistically.

6. *Breaking Painful Patterns*

The faster you learn your lessons the less trauma and drama that you have to incur on your journey. Follow the following five steps to avoid repeating painful lessons.

(1.) Observe your actions while in the experience, like you're watching a movie of your life.

(2.) For clarity, while inside the experience, purify your Temple, with a 7-, 14-, or 21-Day Natural Living or Live Food Cleanse or Juice Fast.

(3.) Study and journal write while cleansing. Ask why you created the experience and what lessons you needed to learn from this creation. Meditate; open up. Get out of your way.

(4.) Listen closely to your inner voice and what you are to do to complete the lesson, so you can finally end the cycle of pain.

(5) Hold on to your Divine Self real tight. Be the captain of your ship and shape your destiny through purity. Don't allow yourself to back track. Follow your inner, spiritual guidance with each step and each breath as you create new patterns to support Divine Living.

7. *We Have A Say So*

The world is screaming; it's in a state of unrest. Look about us. The bombing of schools, businesses and people who inhabit these spaces, with the worldwide rise of AIDS, cancers and all forms of dis-eases and wars, emerging from sea to sea is an indication, a sign if you will, of humanity's collective state of spiritual, emotional and psychological degeneration.

Our defenses are down; our physical immune systems are challenged, which reveals itself in the breakdown and decline of the spirit of a people, leaving us all at risk.

Feel defenseless, powerless and inept? Living in fear of the unknown, of what someone else might do, caught up in somebody else's mad world. Remember, we have a say in what is or what is not to be.

Feel doubt; lost your faith? Your voice is weak or faint, somewhere in the background, where only we hear each other's whispers. We think we cannot effect change, or bring about a healing.

I say, this is not so. As we purify our hearts, our words, our deeds, our consumption, and our toxic attitudes, our natural power shall surface.

I am convinced due to the overwhelming life success of so many who have journeyed on the Heal Thyself Path of Purification, that as we purify our lives, we will experience profound personal and wholistic world wellness. Therefore, everything about us will vibrate in the heights.

As we clean up our personal madness, our past karma (Shai), our voices will be heard. Our thoughts, our words and deeds will cause a profound healing to occur throughout our inner solar system and throughout this planet we call earth.

Put yourself through the test. Clean up your stuff, then speak, and it will be heard. For in truth, we do have a say so!

8. *Learning Through our Crisis*

> In closing, when contemplating with my eldest son, Supa Nova, on the concept of crisis, it came to me that a crisis helps one to move out of his or her toxic creation and while doing so may encourage one to examine the transformative opportunities ahead, those that a crisis reveals.
>
> You have ignored all the signs along the way and the only way that you are going to grow now is to create a crisis. Let us examine the transformative opportunity that a crisis brings.
>
> A crisis arises when we ignore truth. When the crisis comes, calmly examine yourself while you are in the eye of it. Be alert, learn, study, be most watchful, pay close attention, breathe, observe. You will gain much self-knowledge of what you need to do to heal your life. Let us grow from our crisis. Be wise. Allow the crisis to bring forth enlightenment. The crisis forces us to see ourselves, so face it courageously. Ascend, get the lesson and fly. Fly!

Twenty-Three

Testimonial
Declarations

Fasting, through the Heal Thyself Center, has positively changed my life. I've been spiritually, mentally and physically healed and empowered. Tapping into a higher consciousness is now more easily accomplished. My key words are now—*fast and pray.*

Sandra Watson
Director, Family Institute for
Education, Training and Employment
La Guardia Community College, CUNY

In the Khamite legacy, Asar (Osiris), Lord of Regeneration, manifests as Hapi (the river Nile) in its inundation. Periodic inundation, through colonic water cleansing, along with herbal ingestion is the greatest tonic for body and mind. I can attest to the fact that water purification and cleansing as I have experienced at Heal Thyself with Queen Afua has been beneficial and in tune with my Khamitic orientation.

Hru Ankh-Ra Semahj Se Ptah
Sen-ur of the Hetep Ptah Temple

When I went to Queen Afua, my legs were so bad that I could not walk without thick pantihose on. I took the 21-day fast in June and now my legs feel so good. I just rub my legs and thank God and Queen Afua for her help.

Rachel Franklin

When I was a child in Afrika, I dreaded the inner cleansings my mother would treat me to. It is a form of enema called *asa* in my language, Akan of Ghana. However, this treatment prevented my brothers, sisters, and myself from being sick. At the first sign of constipation, headache, stomach ache and other ailments, *asa* was prepared and administered. Unpleasant as it was, that was what kept us bright-eyed, strong and healthy.

Inner cleansings have been an ancient health practice of Afrikans since time immemorial. It was after I started having colon irrigation recently as an adult, that I confirmed this ancient health practice of our ancestors. My eyes are brighter; my sight clearer. I am much healthier all the time. My joints are stronger and I never even catch a cold in this treacherous ecology. My creative level and energy level is so high that I feel reborn.

To the Afrikan, health is inner cleansing and eating healthy. It is law, the law of nature. It is for the birds and the entire animal kingdom. The birds by divine intuition know what seeds and leaves or herbs to pick and digest.

Divine intuition is supreme law. Intestinal cleansing is the guaranteed way to a vibrant, healthy life.

Joe Mensah

Fasting has touched all aspects of my life—the mental, the physical, and the spiritual. Physically, it gave me the opportunity to cleanse my body in preparation for the child I was to conceive. It was not a planned conception, but a truly divine conception. One year to the day I undertook the first of four 21-day fasts, not knowing that the Creator was preparing my body for the birth of another spirit returning, I conceived.

Mentally, fasting has allowed me mental clarity; it removed a lot of mental pollution that clogs us all. It gave me the opportunity to be still and make decisions and choices that had eluded me for years. I finally was able to make the step to economic freedom and the creation of my own law firm with my brother.

Spiritually, it led me further down the path of our divine state. It brought peace, balance, patience, and forgiveness into my heart.

Yet, fasting is as unique an experience as each of us is unique. The particular benefits of a fast may be seen immediately or manifest slowly. A fast is the Creator's tool to bring us to divinity.

Universally, fasting purifies a nation, a world. Remember: Gandhi freed his people with fasting! Peace.

Dianne Ciccone
Esq. (Lawyer)

People cannot believe that I'm 40-years-old; they guess my age to be around 25. I have got more energy than I had when I was 20. A typical day for me starts at 5 a.m. with jogging. I go to work, do all of my house work, laundry and cooking for my family, and go to the gym most evenings. I've also joined two community organizations, something I never was able to find the time or energy for. I no longer bleed every month and the doctor says that my blood count is higher than the average woman's. Every day I thank God for Heal Thyself and I've encouraged all of my friends and family to take advantage of the many benefits this program has to offer.

Judy Shepherd-King

Praise the Lord for Queen Afua and her wonderful staff at Heal Thyself. Richard and I had started the 21-day fast on Sept. 11, 1989 and successfully graduated Oct. 1, 1989. I had the urge to continue the fast, so without a break, I continued the next 21-day fast, further experiencing a renewal and cleansing that I find extremely difficult to verbalize. During all this time, I was receiving regular colonics, steam baths, body massages, following instructions from *Heal Thyself*, drinking large quantities of (purified) water and having full emotional and physical support from my husband.

As the second 21 days began to come to a close, I still had the need to continue—without a break—to a third 21-day fast. During the entire time, I worked every day and had only a 1-day crisis. The only area that I had not followed was the instructions of taking the Sonne seven and nine. For the last seven days, I have taken the Sonne and the results have been awesome. I now understand that cleansing never stops—and we won't stop!

Verran Barter

Before I went to Queen Afua, I was always tired/sleepy. I had no energy. When I decided to go on her 21-day fast, I followed the instructions carefully. Now, I feel great, wonderful. I've never felt better in my life. I have a lot of energy. I feel stronger. My skin looks younger, softer and smoother. I can think clearly, and I understand better. I communicate better with my husband and children. I am more relaxed. I can deal with any type of problem, even those I could not deal with before.

I would like everyone to know that I lost 22 pounds in the course of the fast. I am ready to go on the next 21-day fast. I am even planning on becoming a vegetarian. I have not eaten meat in 6 weeks. Again, I feel wonderful and great. I want to thank the Creator for guiding me and keeping me strong so that I could go on with this fast. I want to thank Queen Afua for helping me get through my fast. While fasting, I prayed to the Most High for healing. I now want to make this my life style forever.

Bayanah Robinson

During the 21-day fasting program, I was able to overcome the desire for drugs. From the first day on the fast, I felt a spiritual healing and physical cleansing unknown to my being. I knew I was truly healed when I could walk past the drug spot and have no desire for some, whereas, prior to the program the need, the desire, and the addiction was ever present.

Thank you. Peace and love.

Name: Withheld by request.

Addicted to drugs for 10 long years

In March 1989, Nazlah began laughing in an uncontrollable manner, which gradually led to trance seizures. At the time, she had a seizure, she was able to hear me; however, she would stare around, play with her fingers, and/or pace back and forth.

After consulting with Queen Afua, she began a nutritional program of solely live food consisting of leafy green salads, freshly squeezed oranges, carrots and beets. In addition, Nazlah was fed fresh fruits, herbs and vitamin supplements.

Approximately 2 months after consulting Queen Afua, the trances ceased.

Nazlah Hudgins

Baker

Illness: Trance Seizures

Length of time: 5 months 5/89-10/89

In 1954, I entered high school. I, then, discovered a blackhead pimple on my right breast. After I squeezed it, it grew into a lump that was, eventually larger than a chicken's egg. Doctors wanted me to have the lump removed, but I kept putting it off because cancer runs in my father's and mother's families. I refused to be "knifed." I did have a cancer test, but I tested negative. I went on praying that this lump would go away someday.

Well, about April 1985, I was introduced to the Heal Thyself Center in Brooklyn, N.Y. This was the beginning of a new life for me. I was introduced to the method of herbal treatment. I first started with the colon cleansing, vitamins, herb teas, exercise and fasting. After 22 months of this method, I was then giving the pack for the breast. The remedy for the breast was to use once daily castor oil, green clay and a hot heating pad, so this could loosen up the lump. Not until the last 2 weeks in July did something happen. One night this lump burst while I was asleep. When I woke up the next morning, I was faced with a new life. This was the greatest experience I have ever felt. It was as if I had released a 40-pound bowling ball from my stomach. I'll always be grateful to the managers of Heal Thyself and to God for this time of my life. Three months of healing.

Thanks.

Sameerah Sabree
Manager
Illness: Tumor on right breast
Length of time 1954-1985
Drugs taken during illness: Herbs

I am very thankful for Heal Thyself because as long as I could remember I have been getting (suffering from) terrible headaches. Since going to them, the headaches have eased up considerably and I have lost weight on the fast program and am continuing to do so. I will continue going to them to receive advice on good eating habits and on my health.

Deborah Jordan
Word Processor
Illness: Overweight/headaches

I am grateful and thankful to the Heal Thyself group for healing my sick body with their prayers and herbal treatments. For 8 years, I suffered with an asthmatic result of the treatment program now I have great physical improvement. I no longer suffer from asthma, high blood pressure or abdominal pains. I am enjoying excellent health.

Angela Terrick
Nurse's Aide and Student
Illness: High Blood Pressure, Asthma, Abdominal pain
Length of time: 8 years

I was sick, disgusted and frustrated with pain month after month, taking painkillers (600 mg. Motrin). I was introduced to Heal Thyself Natural Living Center. During my visit to the Center in September 1985, I underwent a healing process in my body that doctors could not do for me. The pressures and pains I previously suffered had been very intense. But, thanks to a wonderful friend of mine who kept pushing me to go to the Center, I am satisfied with my healing and I am enjoying my life once more. Thanks be to God the Father, and his Son, Jesus Christ; all things are possible. I do hope that more people will start understanding that where doctors fail, Heal Thyself will prevail.

Joan F. Alexander
Telephone Operator
Illness: Menstrual problems
Period: 5 years

In one week or less after starting this fast, all of my arthritis pains were gone. My blood pressure was down to 130/86. Thank God for Heal Thyself Natural Living Center.

Ethyln Olyna Jordan
Clerk
Illness: High Blood Pressure and Arthritis
Period: 20 years

Thema Halstead affirms that she attended the Heal Thyself Center from July 1985 to March 24, 1986. She has received colon therapy (cleansing), nutritional advice and fasting therapy (consultation). During this period, her problems were anemia, enervation, lassitude, cystitis, intestinal gas, and narcolepsy.

Thelma Halstead
Classroom Teacher
Illness: Anemia/anemia-related symptoms
Period: Over a period of years

My healing experience began in 1986. During the first 3-4 weeks, I spent 21 days fasting and cleansing internally, as well as externally. Many of the symptoms of my hormonal imbalance have disappeared: fatigue, dry skin, menstrual problems, headache, lower back pain. I have stopped taking the synthroid and no effects have come up. The herbs I'm taking are correcting the problems that in the past have come up in this situation.

Mary Lee Miller

Teacher

Illness: Hormonal imbalance and fatigue

Length of time: 7 years

Twenty-Four

Epilogue

Purification Oath

Go tell it on the mountains;
go tell it everywhere,
Go tell it on the mountains;
that purification is here,
for I am purified.

    I am purified

       I am purified.

Forgive me,
I will be a sinner no more.
I will not defile the gift
the Creator has bestowed upon me.
I will cleanse and build a body Temple
 of light,
for I am purified.

    I am purified

       I am purified.

Give me the power and strength to release
that which brings about Satanic reaction.
Release me from eating pork, beef, all flesh,
milk, cheese, ice cream, fried foods, and sugar.
Free me from my tumors, my cysts,
my high blood pressure, aches and pains.
Release me from the strong grip of alcohol and drugs.

Free my soul from these desires. For the fall of humankind was ushered in hand-in-hand with these dark tools, and the purpose was destruction.

I cry out, RESURRECTION.
I AM the resurrected.
Creator, help us to turn our backs on darkness
and direct us to the Truth and the Light.
Help us to use the divine tools of inner freedom.
Show us the joys of eating foods made by your hands.
I say "Yes" to fresh fruits, vegetables, sprouts,
whole grains and herbs. For it is said,
"Behold, I have given you every herb-bearing seed which is upon the face of the earth, and every tree, in which is the fruit of a tree yielding seed; to you it shall be for meat."

Let it be known that through the hands of purified souls, bodies and hearts a New Age will be ushered in. Personal, collective and global resurrection begins when we have the power and the faith to accept your divine, unchanging path of purification.

Burdens of envy, pain, hate, anger, rage,
lust, jealously, lack and limitation, today
no more in my life
for I am purified.

    I am purified

    I am purified

Love, joy, abundance, peace, gentleness,
health and wealth are mine,
for I am purified.

    I am purified

    I am purified.

My blessings, my gifts, my hopes,
my dreams, my freedom await me.
Let the heavens and earth rejoice.
I am one of the Chosen Ones,
I am purified.

I am purified
> I am purified.

Let purification ride on wings of air.
Let purification ride on the ocean of Life.
Let purification shine from the blazing sun.
From me to you and you to me.
Yes, go tell it on the mountains.
Go tell it everywhere, that the Creator is here
to let everyone know that fasting,
prayer and purification is the way,
and you must come through the door of purification
to reach God-realization today.
Yes, go tell it on the mountains.
Go tell it everywhere
Rejoice that purification is here
I am purified.
I am purified.

Creator, Neter, Jah, Jehovah, Allah, God Almighty, Krishna, Yahweh, Yeshua, Olódùmarè, I'm home. I've come home to my original purified God-like state.

I am purified.
> I am purified
>> I am purified.

Queen Afua

To all my relations, to the people mentioned herein, to all my clients, my friends, loved ones who have come into my life, and I into theirs.

A Love Poem

We have exchanged healing through the years
I pray our love has grown potent enough to travel
on the winds of our dreams and our realities
I pray our love will be felt in the spirit
even when we are unable to hear or see one another

What peace, what joy we would feel all the time
For this deep love knows no bounds, no limits
I love you, my blood and extended families, for all the
lessons, challenges, and blessings received through you
I love you for being the Creator's co-pilot and for helping
to make, shape and mold me into a healer
Or better still, a vessel of healing
For the Creator is the Grand Master Healer.

We are the vessels that the Holy Spirit (Neter) chooses to
work through if we are but willing to serve.
I love you for helping to make me grow even when
you weren't conscious of your assistance in my evolution.

There is no sadness in my years;
Only tears of joy and understanding
Only bliss: memories of the peace, strength, courage and
soul-searching knowledge we shared.

"No man or woman is an island."
It takes all of us to make you, and all of you to make me.

In Celebration of Our Children

This written word was inspired as I was giving thanks and praises for my children who have sacrificed through their entire life—from birth to now-because of my 24-hour commitment and dedication to my life work, Healing. These words are also in honor to all our children everywhere.

Don't grow up with overt or suppressed anger about your parents. Know that we love you, know that we love you in different ways; so that when you grow from a seed to a tree you will be without resentment, which is illness. You will be a whole, healthy and beautiful tree. Forgive us for all inconsistencies and mistakes and lack of knowledge about parenting. Forgive us for being preoccupied with the world's problems and overwork and overwork and constant worry about your future. I know we will strive to be there for you at times when you need us most. We vow now as parents of the planet to do better, to be more balanced in our decisions about life, and you. Keep this in mind just as you as a child are growing moment by moment into wisdom and understanding. Let us extend patience to one another, parent to child. Let us continue to grow into the greatness of unconditional love: for my love of you is deeper than my soul, and stronger than my own flesh.

We, the Parental Community of the World, vow to guide, love and protect you. We vow to bestow a blessing upon you as you go daily into the world that danger will not befall you. We vow to aid your growth with life-giving and life-sustaining natural foods. We vow to keep your body free from fast food, i.e. fried burgers, soda and other artificial foods that slowly kill and destroy your body, spirit and mind. We will keep you free of flesh foods that makes us sometimes behave in a deadly way, aging us before our time.

We vow to fill you with fresh herbs, vegetables, whole grains, live juices, and sun-ripened foods made by the Creator's hands. Each portion of food you take into your body Temple will not only feed your body, but also your spirit.

We, as Parents of the World, vow not to poison you with violent TV viewing or micro-dinners, or physical abuse in word or deed or glance.

As your mother (Mama), I vow upon your coming to this earth to feed you with breast milk, and comfort and love you so that you will receive the divine nectar that was ordained for you.

As your father (Baba), I vow to be there for you in sickness or health; during life and beyond death.

We vow as parents to be your Nature care practitioners and to use (4) elements to heal you and keep you well from the so-called necessary childhood dis-ease of mumps, measles, chicken pox, ear aches, hyperactivity, colds, fevers and runny noses, and from bad dreams.

We vow to support and nurture the special gifts you come to share with this planet.

We vow to praise all your good deeds, for none are too big or too small. We vow to set good examples so that you can grow strong, confident and stable.

We vow to teach you the spiritual ways so as to repel darkness and draw a life of light, peace and joy unto you.

There is an Afrikan proverb that says, "It takes a whole village to raise a child." My prayer is that through our continued healing of thyself our love enlarges, such that we can receive a continuous and abundant love from one another.

I love you for helping me to write the pages of my life in its many shapes and colors through the eyes of a healer.

Lovingly,

Queen Afua

About the Author

QUEEN AFUA IS A NATIONALLY renowned herbalist, holistic health specialist and founder and co-director of the Heal Thyself Natural Living Center. She is a dedicated healer of women's bodies and souls, who practices from a uniquely Afrocentric, spiritual perspective, and has guided thousands of women and men through the path of purification.

An initiate of the Shrine of Ptah and Chief Khamitic Priestess of Purification in the Temple of Nebt-Het (*an ancient Afrakan order*) in New York City, Queen Afua also is the Founder, Director and Spiritual Guide to the Global Sacred Woman Village Center. She is a certified colon therapist, certified polarity practitioner, Bach Flower therapist, lay midwife, and fasting specialist.

Queen Afua lectures extensively, and has been featured at Downstate Hospital and Brooklyn Hospital where she spoke to a staff of doctors and nurses on the power of holistic medicine; NASA (National Aeronautics and Space Administration); The National Coalition of 100 Black Women; The St. Paul Community Baptist Church, with Pastor Rev. Johnny Ray Youngblood; and at Colleges and Universities throughout the country. She has also served on Essence magazine's holistic Health Practitioners Think Tank. Her message, "Liberation through Purification" has traveled via satellite around the world. Queen Afua has received certificates of appreciation and recognition from:

·The City of Los Angeles and Mark Riley-Thomas, Council member;

- United States Senator, Barbara Boxer, in recognition of her outstanding accomplishments;
- The Rivers Run Deep Institute;
- The City of Philadelphia and Mayor John Street;
- The Senate of Pennsylvania and Shirley M. Kitchen;
- Maxine Waters, Member of Congress, the 35th District, California, in Recognition as a renowned herbalist, natural health and nutrition expert, and in appreciation as author of *Heal Thyself* and *Sacred Woman: Guide to Healing the Feminine Mind, Body and Spirit*;
- The California State Senate in Appreciation of her outstanding service and dedicated commitment toward promoting Public Awareness concerning women's health issues.
- The Wellness of You 2000 Tree of Life Award from Salaam Enterprises, Inc. and Universal Community Homes

The Heal Thyself Natural Healing Method is a loving wellness vehicle that will give a greater number of people the opportunity to heal themselves. For total health, we must accept natural living and fasting as a way of life and as a way of acquiring healthy habits for longevity.

About the Book

Bob Law announced on WWRL Radio Station, August 1990, that Queen Afua was writing a book.

I had not begun to think about writing, but once I got over the shock of this community announcement I looked at this as a spiritual command and message from the Creator to write down my more than twenty-four years of acquired knowledge in Natural Healing and Fasting.

So, I began to write and write and rewrite until August 1991, at which time the first edition of *Heal Thyself for Health and Longevity* was born out of me. It was not an easy birth, but with the help of my editors, the baby is healthy and strong.

In the words of Bob Law, "The future offers each of us significant challenges and opportunities. We can simply repeat our past experiences or we can explore new levels of awareness. We can chart a flight-plan for success."

This book is a manual for the future. It contains ideas that can help each of us reinvent our lives. I believe God wants us to constantly improve on the gifts that He has given us.

BIBLIOGRAPHY

Afrika, Llaila O. *Afrikan Holistic Health*. Brooklyn, New York: A&B Publishers Group. 2002.

_____ . *Nutricide. The Nutritional Destruction of The Black Race*. Brooklyn, New York: A&B Publishers Group. 2002.

Afua, Queen. *Sacred Woman: A Guide to Healing the Feminine Mind, Body and Spirit*. New York: Ballatine Books

Balch, James F., M.D., and Phyllis Balch, C.N.C. *Prescription for Nutritional Healing*. New York: Penguin Putnam.

Budge, E. A. Wallis, *The Book of Coming Forth (Egyptian Book of the Dead*. Brooklyn, New York: A&B Publishers Group.

Ciccone, Diane. *The Heal Thyself Natural Living Cookbook*. Brooklyn, New York: A&B Publishers Group. 1999.

Ehret, Arnold. *Mucusless Diet Healing System*

Gregory, Dick. *Dick Gregory's Natural Diet for Folks Who Eat:Cookin' with Mother Nature*.

Omraam Mikhael Aivanhov *The Yoga of Nutrition*

Pookrum, Jewel. *Vitamins and Minerals from A to Z*. Brooklyn, New York: A&B Publishers Group.

Szekely, Edmund Bordeaux. *The Essene Gospel of Peace*. Book 1 San Diego, CA: Academy Books, 1977

Walker, Norman W. *Colon Health: Key To Vibrant Life*

Duffy, William. *Sugar Blues*. New York: Warners, 1966.

Kulvinskas, Viktaras. *Survival Into the 21st Century*

Heal Thyself Natural Living Center
and
Global Sacred Woman Village Center

Catalog of Products and Services

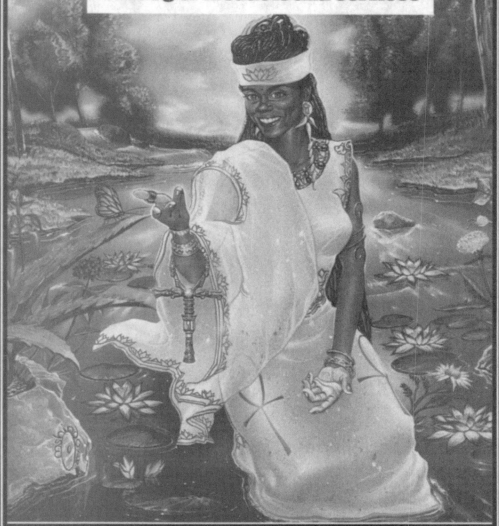

Queen Afua

Founder, Director and CEO

of the

Heal Thyself Natural Living Center

and

Global Sacred Woman Village Center

106 Kingston Avenue

Brooklyn, New York

11213

(718) 221-HEAL

www.QueenAfuaOnline.com

Academy of Higher Learning

Heal Thyself Certification Programs ....

Heal Thyself School of Natural Living ....
 Training Held Spring & Fall Semesters

Heal Thyself 1-Day Fasting Shut-In Facilitator Certificate Training
 As a facilitator, learn how to welcome all levels of health advocates, from
 the novice to the advanced health activist. Teach others how to fast in a
 totally guided, supportive atmosphere. Learn how to inspire others to
 transform into conscious healthy thinkers in just one day of exposure to
 wellness. Learn how to prepare tonics & formulas to support a group's
 purification.

**Heal Thyself 21-Day Fasting and Live Food Cleansing Consultation
Facilitator, Certificate Training** ....
 Teach the Heal Thyself natural living philosophy as way of life to assist one
 to transform from a dis-ease state to a healthy state. Learn how to facilitate
 an individual or a group cleansing and assist rejuvenation of body, mind and
 spirit atonement. Learn how to present the use of fruits, vegetables, juice
 therapy, herbs, clay, oils, exercise, and proper breathing with the use of the
 five elements of nature to Heal Thyself.

Heal Thyself Vegetarian Food Specialist ....

Foods as Medicine Series
 Learn how to prepare delicious, healthy vegetarian foods that rejuvenate,
 purify and heal the body temple. Learn proper food combination, herbs and
 spices, to excite the taste buds. Learn how to prepare whole grains, meatless
 protein green food cuisines and fun-filled deserts. Learn sprouting and
 wheatgrass growing for advanced wellness. Experience vegetarian food
 preparation as a unique style of using food as medicine.

Call for Spring or Fall Certification

Heal Thyself Certificate Facilitator/4 days Hands-on-Intensive /12-Week
Internship

CALL ABOUT SACRED WOMEN INITIATION TRAINING

Heal Thyself/Sacred Woman Wellness Products

Price

01: Green Life Super Nutritional Formula I ....$ 18.00

02: Master Herbal Formula II 18.00

03: Inner Ease Colon Deblocker Formula III..............................10.00

04: Cascara Sagadra Herbal Laxative Tablets IV 7.00

05: Queen Afua's Rejuvenation Clay 8 oz. V 18.00

   Queen Afua's Rejuvenation Clay 4 oz. V.................................12.00

06: Breath of Spring Mucus Decongestor VI 15.00

07: Woman's Life Herbal Formula VIII....................................... 15.00

08: Heal Thyself 21-Day Cleansing Kit........... ....90.00
   Includes 21-Day Supply of Formulas: (3) Formula 1 (3) Formula 2
   (3) Formula 3 (1) Formula 4 (1) Breath of Spring (1) 4 oz. Clay
   (1) Manual (1) Instructional Folder (1) Heal Thyself book.

09 Heal Thyself 7-Day Cleansing Kit ....
   Includes 7-Day Supply of Formulas: (1) Formula 1 (1) Formula 2
   (1) Formula 3 (1) Formula 4 (1) Breath of Spring (1) 4 oz. Clay
   (1) Manual (1) Instructional Folder.

HEAL THYSELF EDUCATION LITERATURE

10: Heal Thyself For Health & Longevity by Queen Afua..........13.00

11: Heal Thyself Natural Living Cookbook by Diane Ciccone ..11.00

HEAL THYSELF AUDIO

12: Heal Thyself Audio 15.00

13: Womb Works Audio Tape...10.00

14: Indwelling Healer Audio Tape 10.00

15: The Great Awakening Audio Tape..10.00

HEAL THYSELF VIDEO

16: Kitchen Power Cooking Class Video 25.00

17: 21-Day Fasting Video Course – 8 hrs. 59.95

18:Sacred Woman: A Guide to Healing the Feminine Body, Mind & Spirit

    Paperback ....16.00 ....hardcover 28.00

19:Dance of the womb Exercise Chart 10.00

20 Sacred Woman T-Shirt 15.00

21:Essential Oil for each Gateway 7.00

22:MAAT feather: small/largesmall....................................4.00 or 12.00

23:Nebt-Het/Ast Sister to Sister Sacred Shawl---raw silk in purple

    or white with gold glyphs ....Call

24:Incense Burner 10.00-20.00

25:Libation Bowl 5.00-10.00

26:Sacred Music Instrument ....Call

27:Stones for each Gateway ....Call

28.We Are What We Eat 15.00

28:Sacred Woman Music CD "Medicine Song" 15.00

29: **Sacred Woman Prayer Card Set**...10.00

30: **Nebt-Het Temple Aromatherapy**... 7.00

Sandalwood/Jasmine/Rosemary/Cinnamon/Eucalyptus/

Lavender/White Rose/Frankincense/Myrrh/Lotus Oil

31: **The Art of Consumption: An informative inspirational video by**

Supa Nova Slom.. **call for price**

32. **Sacred Jewelry from the Studio of PATH –**

Sacred Woman Khermetic wedding bands/Initiation

Rings/Pendants

Call 1(212) 226-8487

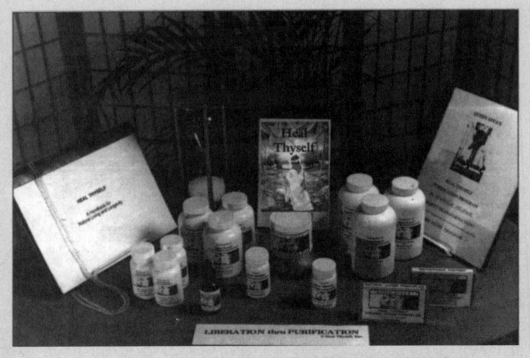

Call and become a certified Heal Thyself Product Distributor

Queen Afua's All Purpose Rejuvenation Clay For Beauty and Wellness

Clay has been used since antiquity in Ancient Egypt for ridding the body of aches and pains and many other afflictions. Our ancestors have used the clay for the beautification of the body Temple. Experience Queen Afua's Rejuvenation Clay in this present age and follow the ancient tradition of our elders by using this "Body Food" to nourish and restore your body temple to balance, beauty and wellness.

Uses of Clay:
Organic facials
Brightens and Whitens Teeth and Gums
Body Wrap or Bath
Bone Rejuvenator
Insect Bites and Scrapes
Softens and Beautifies Hands and Feet
Hair Conditioner
Cover Eye Lids for Eye Restoration

Queen Afua's Rejuvenation Clay 8 oz. jar **18.00**

Queen Afua's Rejuvenation Clay 4 oz. jar **12.00**

7-Day Kit Includes **$90.00**
(1) Green Life Formula 8 oz. (1) Master Herbal Formula 12 oz.
(1) Colon Ease; (1) Herbal Laxative; (1) Breath of Spring;
(1) Rejuvenation Clay 4 oz. (1) Manual; (1) Instructional Folder;

21-Day Kit Includes **$195.00**
(1) Green Life Formula 8 oz. (3) Master Herbal Formula 12 oz.
(3) Colon Ease; (3) Herbal Laxative; (1) Breath of Spring;
(1) Rejuvenation Clay; (1) Manual; (1) Instructional Folder;
(1) *Heal Thyself* book.

For Private Wholistic Wellness Consultation with Queen Afua
Call (718) 221-HEAL

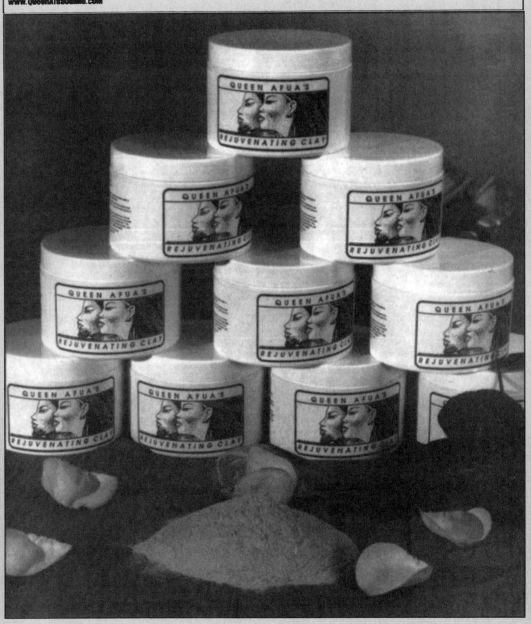

Index

EWorld Inc.
Send for our complete full color catalog today!

Prices subject to change without notice

Mail To: EWorld Inc. - 1609 Main St. - Buffalo - New York - 14209
TEL: (716) 882-1704 FAX: (716)882-1708 EMAIL: eeworldinc@yahoo.com

NAME_____

ADDRESS_____

CITY_____ ST _____ ZIP _____